KV-375-576

Ernest Anthony Azzopardi
Bill McWilliams
Dean Boyce

Gram-negative Burn Wound Infection

A08808

Ernest Anthony Azzopardi
Bill McWilliams
Dean Boyce

Gram-negative Burn Wound Infection

An Evidence Based Approach

LAP LAMBERT Academic Publishing

Impressum/Imprint (nur für Deutschland/ only for Germany)

Bibliografische Information der Deutschen Nationalbibliothek: Die Deutsche Nationalbibliothek verzeichnet diese Publikation in der Deutschen Nationalbibliografie; detaillierte bibliografische Daten sind im Internet über http://dnb.d-nb.de abrufbar.

Alle in diesem Buch genannten Marken und Produktnamen unterliegen warenzeichen-, marken- oder patentrechtlichem Schutz bzw. sind Warenzeichen oder eingetragene Warenzeichen der jeweiligen Inhaber. Die Wiedergabe von Marken, Produktnamen, Gebrauchsnamen, Handelsnamen, Warenbezeichnungen u.s.w. in diesem Werk berechtigt auch ohne besondere Kennzeichnung nicht zu der Annahme, dass solche Namen im Sinne der Warenzeichen- und Markenschutzgesetzgebung als frei zu betrachten wären und daher von jedermann benutzt werden dürften.

Coverbild: www.ingimage.com

Verlag: LAP LAMBERT Academic Publishing GmbH & Co. KG
Dudweiler Landstr. 99, 66123 Saarbrücken, Deutschland
Telefon +49 681 3720-310, Telefax +49 681 3720-3109
Email: info@lap-publishing.com

Herstellung in Deutschland:
Schaltungsdienst Lange o.H.G., Berlin
Books on Demand GmbH, Norderstedt
Reha GmbH, Saarbrücken
Amazon Distribution GmbH, Leipzig
ISBN: 978-3-8383-9025-3

Imprint (only for USA, GB)

Bibliographic information published by the Deutsche Nationalbibliothek: The Deutsche Nationalbibliothek lists this publication in the Deutsche Nationalbibliografie; detailed bibliographic data are available in the Internet at http://dnb.d-nb.de.

Any brand names and product names mentioned in this book are subject to trademark, brand or patent protection and are trademarks or registered trademarks of their respective holders. The use of brand names, product names, common names, trade names, product descriptions etc. even without a particular marking in this works is in no way to be construed to mean that such names may be regarded as unrestricted in respect of trademark and brand protection legislation and could thus be used by anyone.

Cover image: www.ingimage.com

Publisher: LAP LAMBERT Academic Publishing GmbH & Co. KG
Dudweiler Landstr. 99, 66123 Saarbrücken, Germany
Phone +49 681 3720-310, Fax +49 681 3720-3109
Email: info@lap-publishing.com

Printed in the U.S.A.
Printed in the U.K. by (see last page)
ISBN: 978-3-8383-9025-3

Acknowledgments

Few authors have been as fortunate in the generosity of so many established leaders in their field by way of advice and unwavering support. In particular, this work would not have been possible without the steadfast encouragement, gentle direction and endless patience of Professor David W. Thomas at Cardiff University. Gratitude is due to Drs. David Herndon (Galveston, USA) and James Gallagher (NY USA) for their helpful correspondence; to Mr William A. Dickson at the Welsh Centre for Burns & Plastic Surgery in Swansea, UK for his indispensable advice; Mr Srinivasan Iyer (Slough, UK) and Dr Shabnam Iyer (Reading, UK) for his support, and her expert counsel in microbiology. I would also like to express my appreciation to Mr Christopher Khoo (Windsor, UK) who held my hand during darker days, truly a scholar and gentleman.

Heartfelt thanks go to Natalia Nicolaev and the staff at Lambert Academic Publishing for their months of patient suffering; to Ernest Senior and Bernadette for making it all happen. Finally I would like to thank my wife Elayne, for her selfless devotion during months of virtual bereavement until the fruit was borne of this labour of love.

This work is dedicated to our patients, who have always been a source of inspiration, resilience and motivation, our greatest teachers.

Ernest Anthony Patrick Azzopardi MRCSEd MScSurg MD
Cardiff, UK

i

Preface

Burn wound infection has been and remains a major cause of mortality and morbidity in patients who have sustained burn injury. The last few decades have ushered in quantum changes in burn care. Burns Surgeons now perform earlier excision and closure of the burn wound with a combination of autograft, (including cultured cells), allograft or synthetic biological skin products to provide wound cover. But despite these advances in wound management patients still develop wound and systemic sepsis.

This study has identified that the prescribing of antimicrobial therapy has been on an empirical clinically based view, particularly in the early stages when there are no microbiological reports to guide appropriate antibiotic use. It presents a thorough review of the literature to develop the evidence for the aetiological profile, incidence and specific risk factors for Gram negative infection in burn patients.

Ernest Azzopardi's extensive research has allowed an evidence based Gram negative microbiological profile to be defined. It is hoped this will usher change in allowing appropriate antibiotic therapy to be prescribed. Recommendations are made to guide further research. It is augured this will focus the research effort by clinicians and academics alike in targeting novel and effective mechanisms to combat this disease. This review is essential reading for all clinicians involved in Burn Care.

William A Dickson MBE FRCS(Glas) FRCS

Director
The Welsh Centre for Burns and Plastic Surgery, Swansea, UK

Table of Contents

List of Tables

List of Figures

List of Appendices

List of Abbreviations

Abbreviation	Full Text
ABA	American Burns Association (USA)
APACHE score	Acute Physiology and Chronic Health Score
BWI	Burn Wound Infection
CDC	Centre for Disease Control
EBM	Evidence Based Medicine
EM	Electron Microscopy
FSTB	Full Thickness Skin Burns
HAI	Hospital Acquired Infection
ICS	Infection Control Specialist
LOS	Length of Stay
NNIS	National Nosocomial Infection Surveys
NLM	National Library of Medicine
NI	Nosocomial infection
PICO	Patient, Intervention, Control Manoeuvre, Outcome
RSS™	Really Simple Syndicate Feeds
SIRS	Systemic Inflammatory Response Syndrome
TBSA(B)	Total Body Surface Area (Burnt) (%)

Chapter 1: Introduction

Gram-negative burn wound infection significantly increases morbidity mortality (Ansermino and Hemsley 2004; Babik et al. 2008; Church et al. 2006) and cost of care (Chim et al. 2007; Ozkurt et al. 2005). Gram-negative pathogens are responsible for the majority of infections beyond the early post-burn period (Church et al. 2006; Singh et al. 2003). Implication of Gram negative organisms in burn wound infection presents particular challenges to the burn surgeon. Besides the gamut of virulence factors associated with Gram negative pathogens, particular manifestations in burn wounds present particular challenges. Biofilm formation has been demonstrated in burn wound isolates (Harrison-Balestra et al. 2003), reflecting complex resistance strategies against host immunity and antimicrobial therapy (Ceri et al. 1999). Gram-negative micro-organisms also rapidly develop antimicrobial resistance (Clark et al. 2003), and inter-species transference of resistance has been observed. In contrast to Gram-positive infection, Gram-negative infection in burn patients incurs a significantly higher mortality (Mason et al. 1986).

Simultaneously, thermal injury deprives the patient of a major host defence system (Church et al. 2006), skin barrier function (Armour et al. 2007), and provides an exudate rich medium that is ideal for microbial growth (Calum et al. 2009; Edwards-Jones and Greenwood 2003). Severe thermal injury may also create an immunosuppressed state, further favouring bacterial colonisation and infection (Calum *et al* 2009). Several studies have addressed the development of Systemic Inflammatory Response Syndrome (SIRS) a degree of which is present in most thermally injured patients (Dahiya 2009; Huang et al. 2008; Ipaktchi et al. 2006). These clinical considerations distinguish the behaviour of Gram-negative BWI apart from the general population of patients with wounds from other aetiology, (Dougherty and Waxman 1996; Oncul et al. 2002). This limits the applicability of data extrapolated form other populations. Furthermore, these factors alter the classical clinical and biochemical signs of infection in burn patients from the general population making sepsis harder to diagnose. The conclusions of studies addressing Gram-negative infection in the general patient population may not be confidently applied to this specific set of patients. While several independent studies have investigated Gram-negative burn wound infection it is still a major concern that no structured evidence-based evaluation on the aetiology incidence and risk factors of Gram negative burn wound infection has been performed.

1.1 Development of the research question

The structured formulation of an answerable research question was attempted, to enable an effective and relevant literature-retrieval strategy. The PICO format advocated by Strauss et al. (2005) was adopted to formulate this study's questions that are key to efficient, high quality evidence retrieval and evidence based decisions (Ebell 1999; Meyer 2004; Richardson et al. 1995). Table 1, applied to the study's question summarises the key elements of this study process using a modified PICO framework.

Table 1: PICO framework applied to the study question

Frame/ Mapped Semantic Class	Intention
Problem and Population of interest Age; gender; treatment status; disease; symptom	Hospitalised burn wound patients. Adult civilian patients. Aetiology of Gram Negative Burn Wound Infection in this population
Aetiology [intervention] of interest Aetiological Agent of Interest	Gram-negative infection.
Comparator of Interest	Current clinical practice.
Outcome (intended) **Patient Outcome**	Recommendations for clinical practice.

1.1.1 The Population of Interest

Several studies highlighted major differences between burn injury wounds and other types of traumatic wounds (Dougherty and Waxman 1996; Santucci et al. 2003). It was also evident from the literature that civilian and military burn wound injuries may constitute different populations in terms of co-existent aetiology and bacteriological profiles (D'Avignon et al. 2008; Gomez et al.

2009; Kauvar et al. 2006; Miranda et al. 2008). Several authors document differences in the immunological response to burn injury between paediatric and adult populations (Moissenet et al. 2000; Yousefi-Mashouf and Hashemi 2006). Our research in this volume therefore, focuses specifically on hospitalised civilian adult patients with Gram-negative BWI.

1.1.2 Aetiology & Comparator

The PICO frame was modified to include Huang et al.'s (2006) recommendation that underlined the need for the interventional frame to incorporate an aetiological dimension. Hence, the bacteriological profile, incidence and risk factors for Gram-negative infection were included in this frame.

1.1.3 Outcome of Interest

This study is expected to ascertain the aetiological profile, incidence and specific risk factors of Gram-negative burn-wounds infection in hospitalised adult civilian burn patients. This evidence will be used to underscore recommendations informing initial antimicrobial 'best guess' therapy until arrival of the final microbiology results. Other significant outcomes include a set of suggestions for refining current methodological designs to inform future research.

1.2 Research Aim

The focus of this study is determined by the research question that guides the study throughout: On the basis of the best available evidence what are the aetiological profile, incidence and risk factors of Gram-negative burn-wounds infection in hospitalised adult civilian burn patients?

The purpose of this study is therefore to determine aetiological profile, incidence and specific risk factors of Gram-negative burn-wounds infection in hospitalised adult civilian patients though an appraisal, critical analysis and synthesis of current best evidence obtained though a structured literature search. On the basis of this study's outcomes, recommendations will be made to improve local bedside decisions on the initial management of Gram-negative BWI. This study will also contribute to the development of current methodological designs through suggestions for consideration in future research.

1.3 Rationale for the Study

The current knowledge-base on the aetiology of Gram-negative BWI consists of studies from individual burn centres based on the current clinical opinion that each burn centre is characterised by a unique Gram-negative microbiological profile (Agnihotri et al. 2004; Edwards-Jones and Greenwood 2003; Guggenheim et al. 2009; Kaushik et al. 2001; Tredget et al. 2004). However, conclusions of these independent studies tend to vary depending on the methodologies and operational definitions used. Hence, it is unclear whether the results based on these studies are due to unique institutional microbiological profiles or due to differences in the methodological designs, which reflect varying degrees of rigour, generaliseability and validity. Despite the importance of Gram-negative burn wound infection the literature lacks an exhaustive appraisal analysis and synthesis of current best evidence on which the probable aetiology, incidence and risk factors for Gram-negative burn wound infection in contemporary practice can be based.

Such evidence would underpin key clinical decisions that the burns team may need to take in the likely scenario of Gram-negative BWI. Such decisions include the commencement of empirical antibiotics, their continuation until the exact microbiological diagnosis plus susceptibility is available to guide bedside management, and minimisation of risk for acquiring Gram-negative BWI. This would reduce the reported morbidity, mortality and cost of care. Dawes et al. (2005) were emphatic in pointing out that an exhaustive appraisal analysis and synthesis of "best available current and relevant evidence" are essential in timely lifesaving decisions.

From the time of clinical diagnosis and urgent Gram-staining to the arrival of the full microbiology report, the surgeon needs to make a decision on the antimicrobial therapy to be started empirically. During this short time-frame the patient may rapidly become highly systemically unstable. There are currently no evidence-based recommendations founded on robust and valid studies to inform the surgeon as to what the likely Gram negative pathogens are, with which this decision can be informed. Burn patients are particularly prone to sudden systemic embarrassment in the face of infection (Barret et al. 2005; Herndon 1996) necessitating emergent treatment with empirical 'best guess' antimicrobial therapy, until microbiological samples are taken, transferred, processed and returned for bedside use. (Agnihotri et al. 2004). In other instances such as developing countries, such sensitivities may never even be available throughout the infective episode (Komolafe et al. 2003; Ozumba and Jiburum 2000). Such practices may contribute to acquisition of multiple drug resistance, for which Gram-negative pathogens are particularly renowned (Church et al. 2006;

4

Edwards-Jones and Greenwood 2003). Furthermore, severely burnt patients typically experience extended stays in dedicated units (Baker et al. 1996; Herndon 1996). Gram-infection is widely accepted to predominate BWI beyond the early post-burn period, and the moist, serous burn wound surface, with ideal ambient temperatures, provides optimal breeding grounds (Church et al. 2006). It may therefore be argued that exposure to multiple 'best guess antibiotics' during infective episodes may encourage multiple drug resistance (Appelgren et al. 2002). One of the aims of this study is therefore to propose evidence-based recommendations about the likely aetiology of Gram-negative burn wound infection founded on current best evidence.

Various studies have been published about the risks for acquiring wound infection in the general patient population (Flattau et al. 2008; Maragakis and Perl 2008; Mshana et al. 2009; Ram et al. 2000). However, burn patients constitute a separate population in terms of risk factors (Hodle et al. 2006; Weber and McManus 2004) and the evidence concerning risks specific to the acquisition of Gram-negative burn wounds infection remains poorly characterised and controversial.

Furthermore, characterisation of the incidence of Gram-negative BWI is important for epidemiology, burn infection-control and surveillance, allocation of resources and targeting the development of new antibiotics to common Gram-negative agents. Within the last five years, five hundred and six new pharmaceutical products have been approved, of which only six were antimicrobials (Boucher et al. 2009; Nelson 2003; Spellberg et al. 2004).

The rationale behind this study addresses both an urgent clinical requirement and a gap in the literature on Gram-negative burn wound infection. An analysis, appraisal and synthesis of current best evidence about the aetiology incidence and specific risks of Gram-negative BWI serves the purpose of formulating recommendations upon which the burns team may institute clinical decisions at the bed-side. It also contributes to further research in the field through suggestions based on various methodological designs scrutinised in this study. Furthermore, with the dawn of polymer therapeutics, whereby existent antibiotics may be engineered into a specific therapeutic profile, (Duncan 2003) the evidence-bases regarding aetiology and incidence of Gram-negative BWI may identify salient Gram-negative pathogens for future targeting.

1.3.1 Suitability of an Evidence-Based Approach

An evidence based approach integrates the best available research to clinical practice, (Strauss et al. 2005) such that clinical bed-side decisions are based on a robust and valid rationale. It entails a reproducible literature strategy reducing the literature-retrieval bias ubiquitous in preceding studies, after the construction of unambiguous terms of reference. An evidence based approach allows an in-depth appraisal of the literature for methodological rigor, reproducibility, impact, internal validity and applicability (Greenhalgh 2001) which current literature lacks. Application of this methodology to the study adds to the knowledge-base by providing recommendations for clinical practice and future research with a robust, valid foundation through an analysis appraisal and synthesis of the literature (Greenhalgh 2001; Sackett and Rosenberg 1995). Furthermore an evidence-based methodology allows an evaluation of the robustness and validity of the presented evidence regardless of methodological designs. Furthermore this approach is ideal to evaluate the evidence from studies with heterogeneous designs. Sackett and Rosenberg sustain that "conscientious and judicious use of current best evidence" integrates clinical expertise in individual patient scenarios.

Limitations of the Evidence-Based Approach

Although evidence-based research has been rapidly espoused as gold standard (Gray and Meakins 2006), its use is also associated with limitations: publication bias, cost, generaliseability and applicability (Sackett et al. 1996) were aspects of particular concern. Studies may be expensive to perform and publish and funding of studies demonstrating a requirement for products manufactured by industry could pose a threat to the validity of evidence-based research (Strauss et al. 2005). Application of evidence-based recommendations may also be expensive, limiting their applicability to clinical practice. Furthermore, studies demonstrating negative results are less likely to be published (Jadad 1998), which could limit the effectiveness of reproducible search strategies.

1.3.2 Operational Definitions

The following operational definitions have been adopted for the purposes of the study.

Burn Wound: Thermal injury causing a loss of epithelial integrity in the skin

Incidence: The number of new cases of a given disease during a given period in a specified population.

Risk: The quotient of an adverse event and the total number of exposures

Adult: All individuals aged 19 years and upwards

Hospitalised Patients: Any patient admitted to a health care institution primarily for the treatment of a [thermal] injury.

Chapter 2: The Structured Literature Search Strategy

The aim of the literature retrieval strategy was to retrieve a maximum amount of studies on the aetiological profile incidence and risk factors of Gram-negative hospital-acquired burn wound infection in civilian adult patients. The strategy followed was that suggested by Straus et al. (2005) summarised in table 2. Recent surgical practice has favoured a paradigm shift from the traditionalist and routine, towards evidence-based surgery (Gray and Meakins 2006). Furthermore, several authors (Strauss et al. 2005; Wente et al. 2003) underscored the importance of integrating evidence-based surgery to the surgeon's clinical expertise in individual circumstances so that uptake of the evidence-based recommendations is facilitated in actual practice.

Table 2: Conduct of the Literature Review & Critical Appraisal.
Source: Strauss et al. (2005)

STEP 1	Producing an answerable clinical question
STEP 2	Tracking down the evidence with which to answer that question
STEP 3	Critically appraising that evidence for validity impact and applicability
STEP 4	Integrating critical appraisal with clinical expertise- recommendations for practice

2.1 The literature search strategy

The first step in the literature search strategy was to identify search terms that were used in a first generation electronic search, whose results were manually screened for relevance. A second generation search manually refined these results through back-referencing and unpublished/gray literature was sought. An electronic automatic feedback loop was set up to ensure inclusion of the most recent literature. Full reporting of the search strategy increased reproducibility and minimised the risk of database bias.

A combination of free text and Medical Subject Heading (MeSH) terms were used to increase search sensitivity, in accordance to Mayer (2004). MeSH headings were identified using the National Library of Medicine MeSH Descriptor Data Browser (NLM 2009). The selected terms, which are reproduced in table 3, were compared to literature already available to identify synonymous terms and orthographic differences. The resulting terms were used to retrieve the

8

literature relevant to the research questions. A search string was then constructed using Boolean operators. Orthographic permutations are reported in parentheses. Wildcard truncations ($) were used where possible to identify all the terms related to the same stem. A first generation search was electronically conducted, using the OVID-SP ™ and PUBMED™ gateways. The databases searched are listed in table 4.

Table 3: Search Terms Used in the Literature Search

MeSH®	Free text	Limitations
Infect$	Infectious AND disorder	1999-2009
Gram-Negative	Gram AND negative	Articles in English
Hospital-Acquired	drug AND resistance AND multiple [MDR]	Human
Microbiol$	Burn$	Adult
Bacter$	HAI	
Multi-drug AND resistance		
Thermal		
Wound		
Injur$		
Traum$		
Incidence		
Risk		

Table 4: Databases Searched Electronically

Multi-file	Databases
Gateway: OVID SP	
Evidence Based Medicine Reviews	ACP journal club; Database of Abstracts of Reviews of Effects; Cochrane Central register of Controlled Trials; Health Technology Assessments; Cochrane Database of Systematic Reviews; National Health Service Economic Evaluation; Cochrane Methodology Register.
Healthcare Information Service of the British Library	Allied & Contemporary Medicine Database Guide (AMED)
British Nursing Index	BRNI Segment BNIB segment
Exerpta Medica Database (EMBASE)	EMBASE database EMBASE drugs & Pharmacology (EMDP) EMBASE psychiatry reports (EMPS)
National Library of Medicine (NLM)	Index Medicus ® International Nursing Index ® Index to dental literature®
Pre-Medline	The Ovid Medline ® In process & Other Non indexed Citations Database consists of in –process and Pubmed –NOT-Medline records from the NLM
International Pharmaceuticals Abstract Database	International Pharmaceuticals Abstracts database

The results of the electronic search for the first clinical question are illustrated in table 5. The aim of the first generation electronic literature search was to produce maximal retrieval of literature to inform the study question. It was necessary to filter the results to increase specificity of the retrieved literature to this study's question. Hence a number of filtration steps were added to the search using the Boolean 'NOT' connector, in table 5 steps 8 through 14. Step 8 identified the PICO model's weakness to 'capture anatomical relations' reported by Huang et al. (2006). Since the aim of this study relates to skin burn wound infection, the filter keywords in step 8 were introduced.

A second generation search was manually performed through back-referencing the articles retrieved in the electronic search an indexing the journals that appeared frequently in the electronic search. A further 10 articles were retrieved through this method. Finally, in order to include recent references, the electronic database searches were saved online and RSS™ feeds were subscribed to, such that newly published articles fitting the literature search would be received by electronic mail.

The articles retrieved in this fashion were screened for direct relevance to the clinical questions. Through cross referencing the results, 16 papers fulfilled all the inclusion criteria and were included for critical appraisal. These are represented in table 6. The excluded studies together with the reasons for their exclusion are listed in appendix 1.

Table 5: Results of the Electronic Literature Search

no.	Searches	Results
1	((Gram and negative) or Microbiol$ or bacter$ or biol$).mp. [mp=ti, ab, sh, hw, tn, ot, dm, mf, tx, kw, ct, nm, rw]	1874672
2	limit 1 to human	987867
3	limit 2 to yr="1999 –Current	827841
4	infect$ or (infectious and disorder) or (hospital And acquired) or HAI .mp. [mp=ti, ab, sh, hw, tn, ot, dm, mf, tx, kw, ct, nm, rw]	1384510
5	(burn$ or thermal).mp. [mp=ti, ab, sh, hw, tn, ot, dm, mf, tx, kw, ct, nm, rw]	159964
6	4 AND 3 AND 5	2843
7	Remove duplicates from 6	2234
8	7 not CARDI$.mp. not RESP$.mp. not PNEUMON$.mp. not GASTRO$.mp. not ABDOM$.mp. not HEPATO$.mp. not NEUROS$.mp. not UROL$.mp. not BADDER.mp. not URO$.mp. not GENIT$.mp. not VAGIN$.mp. not RENAL.mp. not EYE$.mp. not KERATO$.mp. not OTO$.mp. not RHINO$.mp. not LARYNGO$.mp. not ORTHO$.mp. not MUSCUL$.mp. not VENT$.mp. not UVEO$.mp. not PAROT$.mp. [mp=ti, ot, ab, sh, hw, kw, tn,	870
9	8 not VIROL$.mp. not VIRAL.mp. not RICKETTISA$.mp. not CANDIDA$.mp. not ZOO$.mp. not CYAHAGA.mp. not FUNG$.mp. not PORCIN$.mp. not BOVIN$.mp. not Q.mp. not BURNETTI.mp. not INTRAMEDULLA$.mp. not SPINAL.mp. not ARTHRO$.mp. not TONGUE$.mp. not NORO$.mp. not GUT.mp. not MYCO$.mp. not DENGUE.mp. [mp=ti, ot, ab, sh, hw, kw, tn, dm, mf, tx, ct, nm, rw]	600
10	9 not DRESS$.mp. not MICROARTICULATE.mp. not CUYAHOGA.mp. not STOMA$.mp. not ACNE.mp. not ENDOCARD$.mp. not ACTICOAT$.mp. not XENODERM$.mp. not PHOTO$.mp. not LARVA$.mp. [mp=ti, ot, ab, sh, hw, kw, tn, dm, mf, tx, ct, nm, rw]	470
11	10 not HAEMO$.mp. not RICKETTSI$.mp. not VIRUS.mp. [mp=ti, ot, ab, sh, hw, kw, tn, dm, mf, tx, ct, nm, rw]	430
12	limit 11 to "adult (19 to 44 years)" [Limit not valid in EMBASE,AMED,British Nursing Index,CDSR,ACP Journal Club,DARE,CCTR,CLCMR,IPAB; records were retained]	292
13	12 not MRSA.ti. not METHICILLIN.ti. not GRAM-POSITIVE.ti	274
14	13 not HEMODIAL$.mp. not MILK.mp. not VACUOLE.mp. not FUEL.mp. [mp=ti, ot, ab, sh, hw, kw, tn, dm, mf, tx, ct, nm, rw]	267
15	14 Keep: 8; **16**; 17; 19; 20; 35; 44; 51; 53; 70; 77; 84; 87; 107; 118; 120; 123; 133; 138; 164; 166; 168; 190.	24

Steps 9 through 14 reflect another possible limitation of the PICO frames: difficulty to encode 'fine grained relationship between the frame (Huang et al. 2006). The remaining articles at step 15 were screened for relevance by reviewing the title and abstract.

12

Table 6: Literature Included for Critical Appraisal

	Paper	Design	Aim	Sample
1	(Agnihotri et al. 2004)	Retrospective study	"to determine the bacterial profile and antimicrobial susceptibility of the isolates and to describe the change in trends over the study period."	665
2	Chim et al. (2007)	Retrospective Cohort	"To determine the incidence and cause of nosocomial infections in all patients admitted to our burn intensive care unit (BICU) over a 5-year period"	76
3	(Appelgren et al. 2002)	Prospective	describe a specially designed computer system for the analysis of data, and report the results from the first 3 years of using the system for routine registration of infection in a consecutive series of burn patients.	83
4	(Singh et al. 2003)	Retrospective	"To determine the changing patterns and emerging trends of bacterial isolates and their antimicrobial susceptibilities"	759
5	(Kaushik et al. 2001)	Retrospective cohort	"To analyse the bacterial isolates from the wounds of patients admitted to the Burns Unit and to determine the sensitivity pattern of the commonly cultured organisms'	336
6	(Khorasani et al. 2008)	Prospective Study	"To investigate the profile of micro-organisms and resistance to antimicrobial agents in a tertiary referral burn centre"	113
7	(Komolafe et al. 2003)	Retrospective Study	"To determine the bacterial profile and antibiotic susceptibility pattern of burn isolates at the Queen Elizabeth Central Hospital (QECH), Blantyre"	317
8	(Lari and Alaghehbandan 2000)	Prospective	"To determine nosocomial infections in the Tohid Burn Centre in Tehran, Iran"	582
9	(Silla et al. 2006)	Prospective Clinical Audit	This prospective clinical audit investigated the primary incidence of BWI between the usual burn patients […] and a number of survivors from the Bali bombings during a 3-month audit.	64
10	(Ozumba and Jiburum 2000)	Retrospective Cohort Study	'To document burn wound infection and problems faced by the clinicians'	71
11	Tredget et al. (2004)	Narrative review	An index case of pseudomonal BWI is reported followed by a narrative review of incidence mortality, risks and prognosis	N/A
12	Herruzo et al. (2004)	Narrative Review	A narrative review describing risk two *Acinetobacter baumannii* outbreaks, and risk factors [aim not explicitly stated]	72
13	(Ozkurt et al. 2005)	Case-control arm Retrospective Cohort Arm	"This study was conducted to determine the risk factors for acquisition of imipenem-resistant *Pseudomonas aeruginosa* (IRPA) in the burn unit."	370
14	(Simor et al. 2002)	Case-Control	"To describe the investigation and management of an outbreak due to multiresistant *Acinetobacter baumannii* and to determine risk factors for acquisition of the organism."	247
15	(Wong et al. 2002)	Retrospective	"Multi-resistant *Acinetobacter baumannii* on a burns unit—clinical risk factors and prognosis"	79
16	Wibbenmeyer et al. (2006)	Prospective Cohort Study	'To determine accurate infection rates, risk factors for infection, and the percentage of infections.'	157

The literature search was limited to the last 10 years (August 1999 to present). Current best evidence is usually taken as the last five years. However, expanding the search to ten years enabled inclusion of a volume of unreplicated key papers published in this time period that are still relevant. Furthermore, the isolated and sporadic reports relating to rare and emerging Gram negative pathogens necessitated the removal of temporal limitations on the literature search such that any trends relating to these infrequent infective entities could be suitably analysed. The literature search was limited to literature in the English language. This may have introduced linguistic bias, which is acknowledged in the discussion.

Chapter 3: The Literature Review

3.1 Critical Appraisal

To determine the quality of the primary studies on the aetiological profile incidence and specific risk factors of hospital-acquired Gram-negative burn wound infections in adult civilian patients, a process of critical appraisal (Mayer 2004; Newman and Roberts 2002) was applied to the literature to ascertain that any recommendations of clinical practice would be based on the "best current valid and relevant evidence" (Dawes et al. 2005).

Several tools were available to critically appraise the literature to discern valid and relevant evidence across the span of different qualitative and quantitative methodologies. Rees' (2004) framework of evidence for quantitative research; the Public Health Research Unit (2006) and McMillian and Schumacher's (1997) standards of adequacy for narrative literature reviews were selected on the bases of their rigour and flexibility in applying them to the body of literature retrieved. A particular critical appraisal tool on its own is rarely comprehensive enough to cover each piece of research to the required depth (Rees and Taylor 2001). Polit et al. (2006) argued that elements from multiple tools should be brought to bear on a piece of research such that it could be critiqued to the required depth. The use of multiple validated frameworks increases the validity of critical appraisal and assessment of evidence from a variety of sources and methodologies.

In evidence-based research it is necessary to evaluate studies on the basis of their quality. Phillips et al.'s (2001) "levels of evidence" hierarchy provided this study with a useful stratification-hierarchy framework to reflect the robustness of individual studies utilised to produce graded recommendations. The hierarchy of evidence levels would support the burns clinician reading these recommendations to interpret and analyse the evidence on which the graded recommendations were based (Evans 2003).

3.1.1 Definitions of Burn Wound Infection

The lack of a common definition may render the literature investigating BWI difficult to compare and contrast. A critique of these definitions is therefore essential before embarking on an analysis appraisal and synthesis of the literature on the aetiology incidence and risk factors of Gram-negative BWI in hospitalised adult civilian patients.

Infection in burned patients is harder to diagnose and manifests itself differently. Clinical characteristics of SIRS, common in burned patients (Dahiya 2009; Huang et al. 2008; Ipaktchi et al. 2006), overlap with systemic manifestation of infection (Church et al. 2006) and topical creams alter the appearance of the burned wound (Herndon 1996). Consequently subjective diagnosis of BWI may be difficult and prone to variation between clinicians. Several different operational definitions were retrieved from the literature, underpinned by evidence of varying robustness.

Garner et al. (1988), on behalf of the Centre for Disease Control (CDC) published a list of criteria required for the diagnosis of BWI. The most important criteria were: classical signs of infection in the wound such as early eschar separation and pus; histological exam of burn biopsy or bacteraemia solely attributable to BWI; electron microscopy; and classical systemic signs of infection. These criteria for BWI diagnosis are reproduced in table 7. These criteria were supported by clinical experience rather than underpinned by an appraised and synthesized body of evidence. This is compatible with level-five evidence in Phillips et al.'s (2001) hierarchy. Consensus definitions are expected to be authored by a well-defined multidisciplinary author panel, representing the clinicians expected to apply them in practice. However, burn surgeon and microbiologist input were notably absent. Lack of consideration for changes in clinical practice could have seriously affected applicability. For example, early excision and shower therapy were paradigm shifts already occurring at the time of this review (Barret and Herndon 2003; Mayhall 2003), but Garner et al.'s (1988) review still referred exclusively to early eschar separation, observed only in the days of immersion and delayed excision (Church et al. 2006). Tissue biopsy and electron microscopy, key diagnostic requirements in Garner et al. (1988) kept progressively falling out of use.

Garner et al.'s (1988) criteria are still relevant to this study as they have been used as reference by current research included in this study. They have also been kept unchanged in the latest CDC updated definitions by Horan et al. (2008). It may be argued that a similar critique may be applied to Horan et al.'s (2008) criteria for BWI definition. Studies using these operational definitions may misrepresent the true incidence of BWI in current practice and show lack of sensitivity to other possible manifestations such as those described by Peck et al. (1998).

(Garner et al. 1988) 'one of the following criteria	(Horan et al. 2008) 'One of the following criteria.	Greenhalgh et al. (2001)
1.Change in burn wound appearance or character such as rapid eschar separation or black brown or violaceous discoloration of the eschar or oedema at the wound margin AND histological examination of burns biopsy specimen that shows invasion of organism into adjacent tissue	1.Change in burn wound appearance or character such as rapid eschar separation or black brown or violaceous discoloration of the eschar or oedema at the wound margin AND histological examination of burns biopsy specimen that shows invasion of organism into adjacent tissue	'Wound Colonization. Bacteria present on the wound surface at low concentrations. No invasive infection. Pathologic diagnosis: 105 bacteria/g tissue Wound Infection. Bacteria present in the wound and wound eschar at high concentrations. No invasive infection. Pathologic diagnosis: _105 bacteria/g tissue Invasive Infection. "Presence of pathogens in a burn wound at concentrations sufficient in conjunction with depth, surface area involved and age of patient to cause Suppurative separation of eschar or graft loss, invasion of adjacent unburned tissue or cause the systemic response of sepsis syndrome."
2. change in burn wound appearance or character (as above AND either of • Organism isolated from blood culture in absence of other identifiable infection • Isolation of herpes simplex histological inclusions or viral particles by EM	2. change in burn wound appearance or character (as above AND either of • Organism isolated from blood culture in absence of other identifiable infection • Isolation of herpes simplex histological inclusions or viral particles by EM	1: Objective Diagnosis of BWI A. Quantitative biopsy (can be used to confirm but is not reliable. It may help with identifying the organism) B. Quantitative swab (poor test but may help with identifying organism) C. Tissue histology
3.Burn patient has two of the following: fever >38C) or hypothermia (<36C) hypotension (systolic<90) oliguria (<20ml/hr) hyperglycaemia at previously tolerated dietary carbohydrate level or mental confusion and any of the following • Histology examination of burn biopsy specimen that shows invasion of the organism into adjacent viable tissue • Organism isolated from blood culture • Isolation of HSV Isolation of HSV histological inclusions or viral particles by EM'	3.Burn patient has two of the following: fever >38C) or hypothermia (<36C) hypotension (systolic<90) oliguria (<20ml/hr) hyperglycaemia at previously tolerated dietary carbohydrate level or mental confusion and any of the following • Histology examination of burn biopsy specimen that shows invasion of the organism into adjacent viable tissue • Organism isolated from blood culture • Isolation of HSV Isolation of herpes simplex histological inclusions or viral particles by EM'	2: Subjective Diagnosis of BWI A. Pain, erythema, colour changes B. Unexpected change in the appearance or depth of the wound C. Systemic changes D. Premature separation of burn eschar'

[1] EM= electron microscopy; HSV= Herpes simplex virus

Peck et al. (1998) critiqued Garner et al.'s (1988) definitions as "having neither clinical nor epidemiological value to burn centres and their health care providers" and proposed a revised set of definitions on behalf of the American Burns Association. These were based on different appearances of local wound from cellulitis through to invasive infection and signs of systemic infection. These were also consensus definitions, essentially 'expert opinion.....based on first principles' (Level 5 in Phillips et al. 2001). Peck et al.'s (1998) definitions differed from the preceding attempt in their consideration of contemporary clinical practice and consequent changes in the manifestation of infection. Less importance was allocated to costly and laborious tissue biopsy diagnosis and electron microscopy diagnostic techniques increasing applicability and ease of use. Peck et al. (1998) however, cautioned against strict application of their definitions which would favour specificity at the expense of sensitivity. In fact the authors suggested that clinical discretion should still be applied in diagnosing BWI and hence favoured these criteria for infection control purposes rather than everyday bedside use. Rather than harmonise clinical practice such criteria could lead to discord between data reported by burn clinicians and infection control personnel, as described by Wibbenmeyer et al. (2006). In contrast to Garner et al. (1988) and Horan et al. (2008), the relevance of Peck et al.'s (1998) study derived from input of a multidisciplinary authorship. In contrast to Garner et al. (1988) some literature was cited to support the diagnostic criteria but this was scarce and dated.

This lack of harmonisation of BWI definitions and their relevance to current practice in burn surgery and research were recognised by Greenhalgh et al. (2007) who reported on a consensus conference of the American Burn Association addressing definitions of infection in burn patients. Greenhalgh et al. (2007) classified BWI from colonisation, to local infection and invasive infection. Consensus definitions for sepsis, and SIRS were also presented. Therefore, their definitions were based on invasiveness of the infection, with direct relevance to clinical treatment. Provision of definitions for SIRS within the burnt patient allowed for distinction between the two conditions, which was unclear in Garner et al. (1988), Horan et al. (2008), and Peck et al. (1998). Their consensus definitions were each backed by a 'rationalisation' from a narrative review of the relevant literature. The leap in quality from earlier studies represented by Greenhalgh et al. (2007) is evident from the logical progression of grouped research concepts contained in the rationalisation for each definition. This study succinctly synthesized current concepts in burn pathophysiology, including wound appearance and SIRS, and characterized clinical signs of infection as a departure from the natural burn pathophysiology, rather than normal physiology, increasing clinical relevance. The only difficulty with Greenhalgh et al.'s (2007) study was the absence of explicit critical appraisal and analysis of the evidence on which the definitions are based, which would need to be addressed in future research.

Our study will adopt Greenhalgh et al.'s (2007) criteria for defining BWI because of their relevance to contemporary practice, integration and complementary use of clinical and microbiological criteria and the reported rationalisation process, backed by a synthesis of relevant and current literature. The diagnostic criteria proposed by Garner et al. (1988), Peck et al. (1998) and Horan et al. (2008) would risk under-reporting BWI, and produce conflicting results between literature reported by burn clinicians and data reported by infection control personnel, unless their actual working diagnosis could be reconciled to a more valid standard ensuring comparability of the literature.

3.2 Aetiology & Incidence

3.2.1 Narrative Reviews

This study identified four major reviews which focused on the determination of the aetiological profile and incidence of Gram-negative hospital-acquired BWI in adult civilian patients. Church et al. (2006), Edwards-Jones and Greenwood (2003), Mayhall (2003) and Polavarapu et al. (2008) favoured a narrative approach to address these issues. The narrative reviews generally agreed that pseudomonas infection was the commonest Gram-negative BWI in hospitalised adult civilian patients. However, only Edwards-Jones and Greenwood (2003) and Mayhall (2003) reported incidence rates. These reviews also investigated the literature from different perspectives including the effects of changes in clinical practice on aetiological profiles, and changes in aetiological profiles with time from admission. Several differences could be noted in the conduct of the individual reviews reflecting various discrepancies in their scope, breadth, methodological rigour and validity.

Polavarapu et al. (2008) in their review suggested that *Pseudomonas aeruginosa* is the commonest Gram-negative BWI. Their conclusion is similar to that of the other reviews but lacks methodological rigour. Polavarapu et al. (2008) presented a logical progression of ideas but did not justify why they excluded studies or the time-frame for the literature retrieval, making it difficult to comment on the completeness of the body of literature. An element of retrieval and selection bias (Jadad 1998) weakens the rigour of the review and validity of the results. Furthermore, no inclusion/exclusion criteria were reported. This is aggravated by the inappropriate weighting afforded to minor studies and the exclusion of major preceding studies from the review such as Church et al. (2006) and Edwards-Jones and Greenwood (2003). The omission of previous research reflects a less rigorous methodology casting doubt on the validity of their conclusions. The methodological concerns with Polavarapu et al. (2008) makes it difficult to accept their conclusion based on their review alone. Their conclusions are essentially based on expert opinion compatible with level 5 evidence in Phillips et al.'s (2001) hierarchy. It is still a useful contribution to the investigation of the aetiological profile of Gram-negative BWI in hospitalised civilian adult patients but it needs to be supported and substantiated by other more robust studies.

Church et al.'s (2006) review was more broad-based in its structured aims. The authors adopted a chronological time-based approach to investigate the aetiology and incidence of Gram-negative BWI in hospitalised adult civilian patients. Consequently their literature review was synthesized to reflect the changes in BWI from admission onwards reflecting a logical progression of ideas. *Pseudomonas aeruginosa* infection was once again reported as the commonest Gram-negative BWI but no incidence rate was specified. The literature synthesized by these authors also underscored the predominance of Gram-negative infection beyond the early post-admission period. Church et al. (2006) also synthesized trends in BWI since the pre-early excision and shower therapy era. In concordance to Mayhall et al. (2003), a significant shift was reported since the advent of early excision and shower therapy, providing further credence to the time-limits for this present study's literature search. In contrast to Polavarapu et al.'s (2008) review Church et al. (2006) apportioned more weight to major reviews then to the minor studies. The authors also emphasized the need for standardisation of working definitions for BWI across clinical practice and the research community, to aid BWI reporting, and increase agreement between clinicians.

Mayhall (2003) adopted a comparative approach to the study of BWI. He sustained that the commonest pathogen responsible for Gram-negative hospital-acquired BWI was *Pseudomonas aeruginosa* with a reported incidence rate of 19.3%. He also highlighted that BWI diagnosis is currently based on clinical examination rather than by following any published criteria underscoring the requirement for evidence-based definitions. Like Church et al. (2006), Mayhall's (2003) review illustrated the differences between classical and contemporary management of burn wound infection. Mayhall (2003) particularly emphasized the reduced incidence of infection that was evident from the literature after the change in practice from immersion hydrotherapy to shower therapy. Mayhall (2003) also reported agreement in the literature reviewed, about the predominance

20

of Gram-negative pathogens in BWI with post-burn time. A large citation library was assembled, synthesized on thematically arranged concepts. However, Mayhall's (2003) review indicated a greater degree of depth, illustrated through contrasting conflicting reports, and proposing possibilities for the discrepancies in the results observed. This indicated a higher degree of synthesis and analysis of the literature than preceding reviews. The author also did not stop at published literature but also included gray literature, in the form of personal communication from the CDC illustrating a literature retrieval process that was more complete, increasing the validity of their findings.

One problem with this otherwise exemplary review was that it only considered one study to substantiate the incidence of pseudomonas infection. This contrasts with the extensive bibliography cited for the remainder of the review suggesting that this area of investigation was treated less rigorously than the rest. The review also lacked a critique of the methodological designs evident in Edwards Jones and Greenwood's (2003) review. Although Mayhall's (2003) abstract indicates a focus on the differences between classical and contemporary management of burn wound infection the aims of this review were not clearly set out. As suggested by Mayer (2004) failing to define clinical question does not allow a clear identification of the target population. Consequently, generalisation of this review's results should be viewed with caution. Also, similarly to Polavarapu et al. (2008) and Church et al (2006) a reproducible, literature retrieval process was not reported. Edwards-Jones and Greenwood's (2003) prize-winning study identified new developments within burn wound microbiology. Within this review, *Pseudomonas aeruginosa* was identified as being the single most important Gram negative pathogen to cause BWI in hospitalised adults, with an incidence rate of 20%. Furthermore the authors underscored the importance of the switch from immersion hydrotherapy to shower therapy, and the subsequent decline in BWI. The scope of this research was exhaustive, and thematically organised into sub-themes, constituting secondary aims of which the bacteriological pathogens associated with infection section was of particular relevance. The concept of BWI was explored from a contemporaneous perspective, complementing the reviews by Mayhall et al. (2003) and Church et al. (2006). In comparison to the other reviews this study included a much more extensive bibliography, although the time limit on the search was not specified, possibly introducing the risk of retrieval bias. Similarly to Mayhall et al. (2003), adequate weight was given to major reviews. Furthermore when conflicting evidence was reported, the studies were compared and contrasted allowing the reader to draw informed conclusions. Although this narrative review was comprehensive and methodologically sound, it would still be classified as level five within the levels of evidence framework (Phillips et al. 2001).

The analysis of the four reviews generally informed this study about the position of other scholars in the field. Each review paper explored burn wound infection from different conceptual perspectives. They agreed on the contemporary importance of Gram-negative burn wound infection, and about the predominance of *Pseudomonas aeruginosa* infection within these patients. Agreement was also observed regarding the reduction in BWI following introduction of shower therapy. This contrasts with evidence from Simor et al. (2002) appraised in section x below, who identified communal shower therapy facilities as a significant risk factor for the acquisition of BWI in hospitalised adult civilian patients. The four reviews under consideration enabled an extensive assessment of earlier efforts at completeness and validity. A common concern is the lack of a reproducible literature retrieval strategy, which may have introduced a considerable amount of publication and selection bias, reducing rigour, and validity of the studies. These reviews varied form a poorly referenced and appraised 'journalistic style' reviews as evident in Polavarapu et al. (2008) to the extensive literature synthesis reported by Edwards-Jones and Greenwood's (2003) exemplary literature review. Other concerns include the lack of critique of individual studies, whose results have been accepted at face value, except in Edwards-Jones and Greenwood (2003). The reviews also fail to identify similarities or differences between infection patterns in different international centres. According to Phillips et al.'s (2001) hierarchy of evidence all of these studies are classified as level 5. The lack of an in-depth critical appraisal and analysis showed in these reviews suggests the need for more robust evidence-based research to investigate Gram-negative burn wound infection.

3.2.2 Cohort Studies Addressing the Pattern of Gram-negative Burn Wound Infection in Civilian Adult Hospitalised Burn Wound Patients

Cohort studies formed the majority of the identified literature addressing the bacteriological profile of Gram-negative BWI in hospitalised civilian adults. Although randomised controlled trials (RCTs) would be more suited to investigate causality, an intended pathogen exposure negates their use on ethical grounds. Crombie (2008) suggests that due to these ethical constraints, cohort studies would be the most suitable approach to investigate causality.

Current expert opinion within burn surgery suggests that different burn centres are bacteriologically distinct (Edwards-Jones and Greenwood 2003; Khorasani et al. 2008; Singh et al. 2003). However, this is based on a superficial analysis of the primary studies' results. Several confounding factors could account for these differences, including the effects of delayed admissions from burn/ polytrauma mass incidents, terror attack victims and differences in laboratory reporting accuracy rates. An evidence-based appraisal analysis and synthesis of cohort studies has not yet been reported to validate or refute differences in the incidence and aetiology of Gram-negative BWI in civilian adult hospitalised patients from the primary studies.

3.2.3 Prospective Cohort Studies

To investigate the 'profile of micro-organisms [...] in a tertiary burns referral centre' Khorasani et al. (2008) enrolled 113 adult hospitalised patients over a seven month period into a prospective cohort study. Patients were followed up with 275 burn wound surface swabs and 164 burn tissue biopsies through their hospital stay. *Pseudomonas aeruginosa* was reported as the commonest Gram-negative BWI with an incidence of 14.5%, in concordance to the rest of the literature in table 10. Surprisingly this was the only study not to report Acinetobacter as a common Gram-negative BWI. A 21% incidence of Gram-negative infection could be calculated from their incidences of Gram-negative pathogens in BWI.

Several features reflected a rigorous methodology. Institutional admission criteria and terms of reference were clearly defined and are closely similar to the aims of this study increasing the applicability of Khorasani et al.'s (2008) results. In-depth description of inclusion criteria and baseline demographic characteristics, including age TBSA burn depth, and admission times, synthesized in table ten reduced the risk of introducing confounding factors into the study, in contrast to Kaushik et al. (2001) and Agnihotri et al. (2004). Using a prospective cohort methodology reduced the risk of retrieval bias. Methodological rigour was also increased through a stepwise description of the microbiological technique from sampling to the final result, and through triangulation of data from swabs and tissue cultures. One factor which could have improved the rigour of Khorasani et al.'s (2008) cohort study through reducing the risk of sample bias was randomised sampling rather than a consecutive sample of patients (Jadad 1998). Several aspects of Khorasani et al.'s (2008) design reflected a rigorous data collection. The authors described clinical suspicion of infection as the primary indication for performing surface wound swabbing which was then triangulated to tissue-biopsy results. Triangulation of results with tissue biopsy and clinical diagnosis increased methodological rigour. This methodology also satisfied Greenhalgh et al.'s (2007) criteria for BWI diagnosis increasing comparability. Several authors agree that quantitative modifications of surface wound swabs strongly correlate to infection (Edwards-Jones and Greenwood 2003; Mayhall 2003; Uppal et al. 2007).

One possible limitation of the study was data reporting, as Khorasani et al. (2008) only reported incidence rates for *Pseudomonas aeruginosa*, *Acinetobacter* spp. and *Citrobacter* spp. infection. Although an attempt was made to contact the authors to obtain further incidence data and the occurrence of mixed infection, the correspondence remained unanswered at the time this study was submitted. Availability of this data would have increased comparability and external validity. The qualitative data reported by Khorasani et al. (2008), nevertheless, confirmed data reported by other studies (tables 9 & 10) regarding the commonest BWI Gram-negative pathogens. It would have been interesting to observe the effect which one Citrobacter outbreak would have caused on the overall incidence of other Gram negative pathogens during the time-period under investigation. The features described above concord with a rigorously performed prospective cohort study, level 2b in Phillips et al.'s (2001) hierarchy of evidence.

In their discussion, Khorasani et al. (2008) argued that "[in their study]…characterisation of wound infection and the micro-organisms involved [was] unique", with relevance to this study, an apparently significant lower *Acinetobacter spp.* and increased *Citrobacter spp.* incidence. A closer inspection of their methodology may however explain these differences due to variations in study design, rather than a true shift in the microbiological profile. Several authors in the general literature reported a significantly decreased incidence of Acinetobacter infection in the winter months (Gales et al. 2001; McDonald et al. 1999; Perencevich et al. 2008). It is therefore possible that Khorasani et al.'s (2008) seven month study period may have been influenced by seasonal shift pattern. Furthermore, Abbasi et al. (2006) performed a quality-assessment of microbiology laboratories across Iran and reported that *Citrobacter freundii* was correctly identified in 79.8% of cases. But, the correct identification rate for *Acinetobacter* spp. was significantly lower at only 29.8% therefore, although a critique of Khorasani et al.'s (2008) methodology suggests a rigorous approach, a low accuracy of identification for *Acinetobacter* spp. in local labs may have resulted in methodological bias decreasing the results' validity. This would suggest caution in the applicability of their quantitative results. However, as specific data for the laboratory involved was not available this possible source of bias cannot be securely ascertained. Seasonal variation may have also contributed to Khorasani et al.'s (2008) unusually low *Acinetobacter* spp. incidence rates. The seasonal variation and significantly reduced incidence of Acinetobacter infection over the winter months reported in the general literature (Gales et al. 2001; McDonald et al. 1999; Perencevich et al. 2008) was also likely to account for Khorasani et al.'s (2008) result rather than distinct bacteriological profiles since their study was conducted over six winter months. Thus although individual patient follow-up was adequate, a longer study duration may have contributed to decrease the impact of this potential lurking variable and increase the study's rigour.

Lari and Alaghebandan (2000) prospective cohort study adopted a different methodological approach to determine nosocomial BWI in their local practice. Every admitted burn patient was swabbed immediately post-admission and on days 3, 5 and 7. This data was electronically stored. Swabbing was performed according to an operational definition of BWI based on local practice during the time of the study, which could be reconciled to Greenhalgh et al.'s (Greenhalgh et al. 2007) criteria (see table 13). A step-wise microbiological approach was reported from swabbing to final diagnosis, increasing reproducibility. Lari and Alaghebandan (2000) reported *Pseudomonas aeruginosa*, *Acinetobacter* spp. and *Enterobacteraceae* spp. as the commonest Gram-negative infections (see table 8). The reported incidence of 'Enterobacteraceae' was clarified by correspondence with the authors as being composed of *Enterobacter* species.

The extensive description of the admission criteria for the burn unit and the demographic characteristics of the included patients was provided by Lari and Alaghebandan (2000) which increased their results' applicability, reproducibility and validity (Strauss et al. 2005). Interpretability of the results could have been increased through introducing a control group (simultaneous matched un-infected admissions). The authors reported a 100% catchment for the consecutive sample followed during the study period, and the drop-out rate due to death was

25

documented. This may mitigate for the reported lack of randomisation. Selection bias would however still be a possibility since the study was not blinded. This could have reduced validity.

The stepwise methodological approach in Lari and Alaghebandan's (2000) study design, increased their study's internal validity. The thorough reportage of the validated and referenced microbiological techniques used to identify the isolates increased reproducibility and reflected a rigorous design. The interpretation of wound swab results was based on clinical judgement increasing the relevance of the results and fulfilling Greenhalgh et al.'s (2007) criteria. The authors also reported the time-frame from burn to admission: determining the interval from burn to swab-sampling reduced the confounding influence of time, reported by several authors (Church et al. 2006; Edwards-Jones and Greenwood 2003). However, patients referred from other burn centres, representing delayed admission, could still present a source of confounding variables. A critical appraisal of Lari and Alaghehbandan's (2000) study therefore suggests that this evidence is in keeping with level-3b in Phillips et al.'s (2001) hierarchy of evidence. The 30-month duration of the study would exclude seasonal variation that may have acted as a confounding factor in Khorasani et al.'s (2008) design. Lari and Alaghebandan (2000) investigated primary incidence of BWI over the first week post-admission. In contrast other studies followed patients from admission to discharge or death. While this reduced the risk of data duplication that could have skewed other studies' results, it also meant that direct comparison to other studies could not be confidently performed. Hence confining the duration of the study to one week per patient may have limited the applicability of the results to a reflection on the incidence of Gram-negative BWI over the first post-admission week at the authors' centre.

This study was the only one to report blanket antibiotic coverage, although Lari and Alaghebandan (2000) justified this practice in the local circumstances. This study investigated incidence over the firs post-burn week in contrast to the other studies. Therefore although the available data reported by Lari and Alaghebandan (2000) suggests that the Gram-negative BWI profile at their institution was concordant to the other studies in Table 16 this could not be confidently pooled to other data in the box whisker plot (fig 2). Furthermore, in view of the findings of Abbasi et al. (2006) and Khorasani et al.'s (2008) the identification of significant rates of *Acinetobacter* spp. BWI appears to be a significant finding.

In contrast to the other studies appraised so far, Appelgren et al. (2002) intended to describe a computer system for BWI data analysis. A number of secondary aims were reported including reporting on the incidence and possible risk factors of BWI in adult burnt hospitalised patients at the authors' institution. To achieve this, 233 consecutive patients were followed prospectively from admission to discharge or death over a three year period. BWI distinguished between the study sample (83 patients) and controls. With the exception of *E. coli* and proteus, Appelgren et al.'s (2002) results demonstrate qualitative concordance to the rest of the studies illustrated in table nine. Although not directly reported by the authors, a Gram-negative BWI infection rate of 31% and a 37.5% mixed infection rate could also be derived from this study.

An appraisal of the evidence underpinning these results illustrated a robust and reproducible methodology. Credence to the validity of Appelgren et al.'s (2002) results is derived from the rigorously followed operationalised definitions in use at the authors' institution, an analysis of which indicated concordance to Greenhalgh et al.'s (2007) criteria for BWI diagnosis. A detailed description of institutional policy at the Karolinska Institute where the study was performed further enhanced comparability to other papers and practice and applicability. Validated microbiological identification techniques were cited increasing reproducibility. Chi-squared test was used to analysis basic demographic details between infected and non-infected patients, to minimise the risk of confounding factors influencing the results. Use of chi-squared was appropriate to the categorical data considered (infected versus uninfected and demographic /burn characteristics), while reported p values increased reproducibility. Yates' test was used to prevent overestimation of significance. Use of Yates' test suggests a rigorous approach although it risks being over conservative (Sokal and Rohlf 1981).

Clearly, Appelgren et al.'s (2002) design indicates a robust methodological design, compatible with a well-conducted prospective cohort study (Level 2b in Phillips et al., 2001). In contrast to all the other papers, follow-up was performed once per week, with one wound swab per 5% burned surface area. Excellent correlation between swab results and actual significance of infection was achieved by combined infection control/ burn surgery ward-round while any diagnostic doubt was clarified by consensus between the burn surgeon and microbiologist, increasing the study's rigour. This may have reduced the reporting bias that may be introduced when burn surgeons and ICS staff operate independently, as illustrated by Wibbenmeyer et al. (2006). The sample's attrition rate was well defined, and a 100% follow-up was reported, until discharge or death. One possible limitation of the study was lack of blinding, however, it could be argued that the possibility of retrieval bias was mitigated by the automated data entry and strict protocol described.

Appelgren et al.'s (2002) results inform this study in several ways. In concordance to the literature, BWI with *Pseudomonas aeruginosa*, *Acinetobacter* spp. *Klebsiella* spp. and *Enterobacter* spp. were reported as the commonest Gram negative BWI. Interestingly however, no *E. coli* infection was reported. According to Greenwood et al. (2002) *E. coli* is strongly associated to faecal contamination, and it may be argued that the absence of such infection is the result of the stringent infection control practices reported by Appelgren et al. (2002). Appelgren et al. (2002) also reported their study to be the first European study investigating the long term infection incidence in a burn unit, emphasizing the need for further research in this area. In their conclusions the authors emphasized the need for standardised and applicable criteria for BWI definition.

A further prospective cohort study by Chim et al. (2007) studied 57 adult civilians admitted to a burn unit over 5 years to study the incidence and explore the cause infections in burn patients. Chim et al. (2007) found a BWI infection rate of 29.5%, with *Acinetobacter* being the commonest reported organism, in contrast to the other literature, although the commonest Gram-negative pathogens were qualitatively similar to the other papers included in this study. Like Appelgren et al. (2002) and Lari and Alaghebandan (2000), background characteristics of the cohort studied were extensively reported and compared to non-infected patients (control) admitted during the same period. Microbiological analysis was performed with validated and referenced methods, increasing reproducibility, while re-swabbing at five-day intervals until death or discharge reflected adequate follow-up. Although Chim et al. (2007) reported that they applied the 'standard CDC criteria' of Garner et al.(1988) their study design actually revealed that any patients with clinical signs of infection beyond 48 hours were included as nosocomial BWI. These were related to burn wound swabs that were being taken every 5 days in keeping with Greenhalgh et al.'s (2007) definitions.

Student' T-test with (p<0.5) was used to compare infected to non-infected patients, reducing the risk of confounding factors between groups, increasing internal validity. This test is robust to small departures from normality (Swinscow and Campbell 2002) rendering it more suitable for a small sample size of 57, comparing categorical to quantitative data.

The main findings of this paper, illustrated in table 10 appear to be backed by a robust methodology in keeping with level 3 evidence (Phillips et al. 2001). Although the same Gram-negative organisms are reported for BWI as the other literature appraised, the incidence of each infection would appear to be different. Particularly, this is the only prospective cohort study which reported Acinetobacter as being the commonest Gram-negative BWI, and the commonest BWI overall. Chim et al. (2007)

suggested that the result could be explained by the fact that Acinetobacter is endemic to tropical climates typical of Hong Kong where this study was performed. This would be concordant to the high incidence of *Acinetobacter* spp. BWI in some studies from tropical climes, such as Perth, Australia (Silla et al. 2006) but counter to the results reported by Singh et al. (2003) and Agnihotri et al. (2004). Another possible explanation for these results could be that during their period of study Chim et al. (2007) treated patients from the Jakarta-Marriot Hotel Bombing disaster of 5 August 2003. A similar aetiological pattern was reported by Silla et al. (2006). The latter admitted patients from the Bali Bombings of 12 October 2002 during the course of their own investigation and reported Acinetobacter as the commonest BWI.

Table 8:

Incidence of Gram-Negative Infection in BWI from Prospective Cohort Studies (primary data)

Study	Incidence of Gram negative BWI	Pseudomonas aeruginosa	Acinetobacter baumanni	Klebsiella spp.	Enterobacter	E.coli	Proteus
Appelgren et al. (2002)	31%	25.2%	2.8%	7.4%	9.3%	ND	ND
Chim et al. (2007)	29.5%	19.1%	23.4%	8.5%	10.6%	2.1%	2.1%
Khorasani et al. (2008)	21%	14.5%	ND	ND	ND	ND	ND
Lari & Alaghebandan (2000)*	56%	65.45%	11.5%	ND	3.5%**	ND	ND

	Table 9: Study Summary for Prospective Cohort Studies			
	Khorasani et al. (2008)	Lari & Alaghebandan (2000)	Appelgren et al. (2002)	Chim et al. (2007)
Incl. criteria	Aged >10 years, with PTSB or FTSB burns, were included. From 09/2006 to 03/2007 Admitted for >48 hrs	Adult; >10% TBSA or >2% FTSB Over 18 months' study period Admitted for >48 hrs	[from text] cohort included adult; see baseline characteristics Over 3 years study period	Over study period: 06/2001 to 07/2006 Admitted for >48 hrs
Policy	Early Excision & Graft Immediate admission No antibx prophylaxis	Early Excision & Graft Antibx Prophylaxis if TBSA>20%Iimmediate admission	Early Excision & Graft No prophylaxis	Early Excision & Graft No prophylaxis
Sample	113 consecutive pts	582 consecutive pts	233 consecutive pts over 3 years. 83 cohort BWI vs. non-infected control	57 pts over 5 years
Baseline char.	Baseline characteristics Age (m)=35 Cause(mode)=flame TBSA(mode)= >20	Baseline characteristics Age (m)=35 Cause(mode)=flame TBSA(mode)= >30	Baseline characteristics for cohort Age (m) = 50 Cause (mode) flame TBSA (mode) = 10% Depth (mode) = FTSB	Baseline characteristics for cohort Age (m) = 38 Cause (mode) flame TBSA (mode) = 43% Depth (mode) = FTSB
Design	Prospective Unmatched	Prospective Unmatched	Prospective cohort study with controls	Prospective Unmatched
Data Coll.	275 Semi quantitative wound swabs Triangulated with 164 tissue biopsy	1410 wound swab samples from 582 pts	Surface swabs from each 5% TBSA related to infection.	Surface swabs on admission & repeated every 5 days
Follow up	Each pt followed until death or discharge	Each pt followed until wound healed	Each pt followed for 1 week	Each pt followed until death or discharge
Statistics	Descriptive statistics use to synthesize incidence data & bacterial profiles			
			Chi Squared with Yates' correction to match cohort & control, & associations to BWI	Student's test to compare infected vs. non-infected pts.
Hierarchy	Evidence compatible with level 2b in Phillips et al. (2001)	Evidence compatible with level 3 in Phillips et al. (2001)	Evidence compatible with level 2b in Phillips et al. (2001)	Evidence compatible with level 3 in Phillips et al. (2001)

Both Agnihotri et al. (2004) and Kaushik et al. (2001) investigated bacteriological profiles of BWI at their institution. Although Agnihotri focused specifically on aerobic isolates, it was noted that both studies were performed at the same institution over an overlapping time-frame and were therefore appraised together. In actual fact, an in-depth appraisal of these two studies revealed strikingly similar results, but a noticeable difference in the methodological rigour and validity of the evidence.

Both studies retrospectively retrieved wound surface swabs during the study periods. These studies concurred about *Pseudomonas aeruginosa* as the commonest Gram-negative pathogen, and about the majority of their isolates being mono-microbial, in concordance to the rest of the literature. However table 10 illustrates that from then onwards their results appeared to discord. Actually, Kaushik et al. (2001) reported a similar incidence of *Pseudomonas* spp. Klebsiella and *E. coli* to Agnihotri et al. (2004). However they pooled all the other data into an "other organisms" category, accounting for 12.5% of infections. This reported Figure is strikingly similar to the sum total of *Acinetobacter* spp. and *Enterobacter* spp. reported by Agnihotri et al. (2004), with the difference in totals plausibly referring to the anaerobes excluded by Agnihotri et al. (2004). These factors point to concordance of the true data despite the apparent reported differences.

Table 10: Analysis of incidences from Agnihotri et al. (2004) and Kaushik et al. (2001)

Incidence of:	Mixed Infection	*Pseudomonas aeruginosa* (%)	*Acineto-bacter* spp. (%)	*Klebsiella* spp. (%)	*Enterobacter* spp. (%)	*E.coli* (%)	*Proteus* spp. (%)
Paper							
Agnihotri et al. (2004)	13%	54.1	ND	3.5	ND	2.6	2.6
Kaushik et al. (2001)	9.2%	58.9	7.2	3.9	3.9	ND	3.3

The two studies however, varied in their methodological rigour. Both Agnihotri et al. (2004) and Kaushik et al. (2001) reported the time-frame defining their consecutive sample of patients. However in both cases, the study sample was only broadly described as a consecutive sample of patients over the study period at one institution. This failure to exhaustively describe their study sample reflects poor methodological design (Crombie 2008; Phillips et al. 2001). Similarly it risked the introduction of lurking variables affecting the validity of their conclusions, (Strauss et al. 2005) and limited applicability of the results (Mayer 2004). However, it may be argued that the authors reported a 100% catchment rate of the intended population being studied according to their terms of reference, rather than a study sample, mitigating the potential threats to validity of confounding factors and sampling bias. Agnihotri et al. (2004) reported follow-up by repeat wound surface swabbing until death or discharge. New data was only added as a separate infection if a change in infecting micro-organism was noted, reducing the risk of data duplication which was a possibility in Kaushik et al.'s (2001) study.

The two studies also varied in the rigour of their data collection. Only Agnihotri et al. (2004) reported validated standardised culture methods for identifying isolates. It could be argued that since both studies were performed at the same institution during an overlapping time-period the same isolation methodology could be assumed. However neither paper reported the institutional policy for microbial isolation. Thus, this assumption between the two separate research teams would be inappropriate. The lack of data regarding microbiological identification, and data-handling including de-duplication opened Kaushik et al.'s (2001) study to the threats of methodological, observer and reporting bias.

Agnihotri et al. (2004) and Kaushik et al. (2001) both reported similar qualitative data, and a comparable incidence of poly-microbial isolates, which is also concordant to the rest of the analysed literature. Appelgren et al.'s (2002) study referred to the tendency of microbiology reports to omit isolated pathogens traditionally regarded as contaminants/commensals. Semi-quantitative identification through wound swabs using their cited reference procedures (Forbes et al. 1998) also concorded with Greenhalgh et al.'s (2007) BWI diagnostic criteria. Within this context it may be argued that Agnihotri et al.'s (2004) results regarding polymicrobial isolates was more rigorous, due to the citing of a standardised microbiological isolation technique.

33

The evidence therefore suggests that Agnihotri et al.'s (2004) methodology was underpinned by a stepwise reproducible methodology. They reported their results against validated referenced and published isolation techniques, included an exhaustive follow-up and reported on a study sample double that of Kaushik et al.'s (2001). However the dearth of information defining their study sample means that their conclusions can be only admitted as level-four evidence in Phillips et al.'s (2001) hierarchy. The evidence also suggests that Kaushik et al.'s (2001; 2001) results duplicate those of Agnihotri et al. (2004). Their value would be to support and clarify the latter's results given the identical institution and overlapping study period. The threats to validity illustrated by a critical appraisal of Kaushik et al. (2001) preclude its suitability as evidence-base for recommendations, and would only be compatible with level 4- evidence (Phillips et al. 2001).

In clinical practice the usual turnaround time from swab to result may take up to 48 hours (Agnihotri et al. 2004; Appelgren et al. 2002) during which 'best guess treatment' is usually the norm. Ozumba et al. (2000) and Komolafe et al. (2003) illustrated this situation at the extreme end of the spectrum where lack of technical expertise, and poverty may mean that microbiological analysis may never be available in the course of burn wound infection. In these scenarios, evidence-based recommendations grounded in an appraisal analysis and synthesis of the literature may inform the clinician on the likeliest pathogen. Clinical treatment decisions could then be based on the likeliest aetiological profile based on local sensitivities.

Ozumba et al. (2000) investigated 71 patients over 5 years while Komolafe et al. (2003) reported on 317 patients over 6 years. Patients were followed forward in time from a historical point (admission), a methodology consistent with a retrospective cohort approach. An opportunistic sample was described. Inclusion in the study was based on availability of data rather than randomised sampling. Although the authors cited local conditions of abject poverty, low compliance and poor education to justify their criteria this could have introduced selection bias reducing rigour. Another threat to validity stems from the non-blinding of the investigators which could have introduced ascertainment bias (Jadad 1998).

The long period over which these two studies took place (5-6 years) eliminated the possibility of seasonal variation that may have influenced results (Chim et al. 2007). Ozumba et al.

34

(2000) clearly defined the post-burn interval at which the burns were swabbed, reducing the confounding effect of time on the aetiological profile of BWI reported by Church et al. (2006) Edwards-Jones & Laing (2003) and Mayhall (2003). Ozumba et al. (2000) also cited validated microbiological identification techniques that were used, increasing methodological reproducibility and rigour, in contrast to Komolafe et al. (2003). Due to the threats to rigour and validity arising from the risk of sampling, observer and ascertainment bias, and the risk of confounding factors, it would be difficult to include quantitative data from these studies as evidence-bases for recommendations. It is striking that the qualitative Gram-negative profiles reported by both papers were in keeping to the rest of the literature. It would be tempting to disregard any evidence presented from these level 4 studies (Phillips et al. 2001). However, the authors fully acknowledged their limitations as the best possible in the local circumstances. Furthermore, the dearth of literature from the African continent on the bacteriological profile of Gram-negative BWI in hospitalised civilian adults renders the evidence gathered from these studies as 'current best' justifying their inclusion.

Wibbenmeyer et al. (2006) compared nosocomial infection rates diagnosed by burn physicians to infection control practitioners. A cohort sample of 157 patients was followed over one year and compared to controls for evidence of BWI. Rates of agreement were compared between diagnostic methods used by burn surgeons and infection control personnel. Interestingly, this study found that although burn surgeons 'sought' to use Peck's (1998) criteria, BWI was actually diagnosed based on clinical judgement. Only a 70% agreement rate was found when compared to data reported by infection control specialists who strictly adhered to Peck's (1998) criteria and CDC definitions (Garner et al. 1988). *Pseudomonas* spp. infection was also reported as the commonest BWI at the study institution. Several features indicate a rigorous methodology including explicit definition of the study sample (157 consecutive patients admitted to the study institution; fulfilling Horan et al.'s (2008) HAI definitions); the study period (one year); inclusion criteria for the study cohort and burn unit treatment policy (early excision and grafting and shower therapy), increasing reproducibility. Clinical diagnosis was augmented by correlation to surface wound swabbing, both included in Greenhalgh et al.'s (2007) diagnostic requirements, increasing comparability. Training of data collectors decreased the risk of inter-observer variability, increasing reproducibility and methodological rigour. However blinding the same researchers to the study outcomes would have reduced the risk of ascertainment bias, which could have reduced internal validity. Strict adherence to the operational definitions was reported

35

increasing reproducibility. Furthermore, background characteristics between sample and control groups were thoroughly reported and compared diminishing the risk of confounding factor influences. These reported factors reflected a rigorous study and increased internal validity. Wibbenmeyer et al. (2006) argued that common BWI definitions would decrease misreporting of BWI incidence rates, and could also decrease antibiotic over prescribing. These recommendations were backed by a robust prospective cohort methodology compatible with level 2b evidence.

3.2.5 Case-Control Studies

Retrospective comparison of a sample of isolates to a control sample from a preceding time-frame would allow comparison of the changes occurring in Gram-negative bacteriological profiles over time (Mayer 2004; Strauss et al. 2005). Singh et al. (2003 pp. 129) adopted this approach in order to investigate whether there were "changing patterns "and "emerging trends of bacterial isolates." The authors therefore compared two five-year periods of burn wound isolates to determine whether exposure to selection pressures during that time-frame would result in significant bacterial profile shifts. A total 759 consecutive isolates from 1997 to 2002 were retrospectively retrieved from patients' case notes and lab data, and compared to a similar control over the preceding five year period. Although no major shift in bacterial profiles was reported, an application of Chi squared tests found a significant difference in the infections caused by *Acinetobacter* spp., *Proteus* spp. and *E. coli* species, prompting the authors to recommend routine bacteriological profiling to aid decision making and prevent emergence of resistant strains. Several features in the methodological design reflect a rigorous approach. Repeat isolates from each individual were de-duplicated to avoid skewing the results, unless new infections were reported. The control group was selected from the same hospital, and no change in burn admission or management criteria were reported during the study period. Data collection of isolates for both case and control time frame were analysed using the same transport and isolation techniques in the same diagnostic labs increasing comparability. These factors reduced the likelihood of confounder factors such as observer bias. The laboratory identification methodology used (Forbes et al. 1998) satisfied Greenhalgh's (2007) diagnostic criteria for BWI, and increased methodological rigour.

Chi squared tests were appropriately applied to test for significant differences between distributions of categorical variables, with plausibly normally distributed data. P-values (p<0.05) were reported which, as suggested Swinscow and Campbell, (2002) increase interpretability of the results reported. Furthermore the authors reported inclusion of a consecutive sample of all patients in the case and control time frame. This comprehensive design may have reduced the potential for retrieval bias that according to Crombie (2008) and Greenhalgh (2001) is common in case-control studies.

Singh et al.'s (2003) cases and controls were not explicitly defined in terms of co-morbidity. This could have introduced confounding factors such as variable total burn surface patterns, and invasive devices / procedures which according to Wibbenmeyer et al. (2006) are significantly associated with increased nosocomial infection rates in burn patients, possibly reducing internal validity. The risk of non-equivalence between case and control increases the possibility of type one error. These concerns qualify this study as level 4 in Phillips et al. (2001). However, the main thrust of this study was the identification of bacterial profile at the authors' institution. Despite the possible biases and confounding influences it is still surprising that the clearly presented data did demonstrate a similar microbiological profile to other articles in the field.

Evidence presented by Singh et al. (2003) informs this study through reporting qualitatively little change between two consecutive five year periods, although quantitatively, *Klebsiella* incidence was reported to increase at the expense of a decreased incidence of *Pseudomonas* and *Acinetobacter*. In keeping with the rest of the literature, the majority of isolates were single although a substantial amount of mixed isolates (40%) were reported.

3.2.6 Audit Reports

The literature appraised in this study reported concordance on the common Gram-negative pathogens causing BWI, although the incidences of the different Gram negative pathogens reflected some variation between different centres. One possible reason may be the different co-aetiologies presenting with the burn patient such as co-existent poly-trauma and delayed admission. The occurrence of the Bali terrorist attacks of 12 October 2002 occurred during Silla et al.'s (2006) prospective audit, presenting an opportunity to contrast this cohort to 'routine' burn wound admissions.

Silla et al. (2006) performed a comparative prospective audit 'to investigate the incidence of local burn wound infection'. Over three months, 59 patients (of whom 22 were referred from the Bali episode) were investigated for initial infective episodes. In keeping with a rigorous approach admission criteria for the institution were extensively described, indicating exhaustive infection control practices similar to those reported by Appelgren et al. (2002). Peck et al.'s (1998) criteria for BWI were applied to define hospital acquired infections, while the background and demographic features were extensively reported, increasing reproducibility, and applicability of the results to this study. This also enabled comparability to the Bali blast sample which served as a comparative control. In both cases, these were reported as civilian adult hospitalised patients enabling comparability. However Silla et al. (2006) reported significant delays in patient transfer, concomitant mechanisms of injury and a much higher TBSA as features distinguishing the Bali group from the 'routine admissions'. Further evidence of this paper's rigorous approach was the used of a trial pilot study which reduced the possibility of intra/inters observer variation and use of validated and referenced microbiological identification technique, increasing methodological reproducibility.

Silla et al.(2006) limited their audit to the initial infective episode during the length of stay of the patients. Although this methodology would not allow comparison to the rest of the retrieved literature which examined incidence rates for any new infective episode during the entire study period, the comparative nature of Silla et al.'s (2006) study identified significant differences between burn patients with coexistent poly-trauma and delayed referral. A chi squared test was used to analyse differences in the initial infective episodes between the cohort and control sample, with a reported $p<0.05$. Chi-squared is suitable to analyse categorical variable distribution between samples, however, given the small sample sizes used by Silla et al.(2006) using Yates' test to prevent overestimation of significance for small data would have reduced the possibility of a type two error increasing rigour.

Silla et al.(2006) reported a significant difference in the incidence of primary infection between 'routine' admissions and Bali Blast victims, including infection with *Acinetobacter* spp. Silla et al.'s (2006) paper reported a scenario analogous to Chim et al. (2007) who included data from the Jakarta Marriot Hotel blast incident. However, Chim et al. (2007) did not differentiate this data from 'routine' admissions. It may therefore be argued that this observation could explain the conclusions of Chim et al. (2007) who reported *Acinetobacter*

38

spp. as the commonest Gram negative BWI (see **Error! Reference source not found.**).

Silla et al. (2006) proposed their study as a comparative prospective audit, and recommendations were made conforming to a quality improvement process, based on the results. These include the necessity for infection surveillance, patient isolation. However, given the follow-up of a well-defined and matched cohort of patients in time it may be argued that parts of their study design reflect a close similarity to a rigorously conducted prospective matched cohort study. The evidence presented would therefore be in keeping with level 2b in Phillips et al.'s (2001) hierarchy of evidence framework. This would add credence to their recommendations for reviewed BWI definitions both for clinical practice and surveillance purposes.

3.2.7 Data from Other Sources

Current advice from the British Association of Antimicrobial Chemotherapy website (BSAC 2009) regarding aetiology of burn wound infection suggests a number of potential organisms that are responsible for the aetiology of burn wound infection. This is followed by a suggested algorithm for antimicrobial management based on typical sensitivities of the organisms considered. No citation is reported for this data, which would, according to Philips et al. (2001) be considered as level five evidence. However this would be an excellent medium to cross the divide between current best evidence and local clinical practice. It would be interesting to observe an application of current best evidence to this website whereby Gram-negative organisms reported as common causes of BWI by routine pooled screening would be published. Decisions regarding antimicrobial sensitivities to these organisms could then be then taken locally depending on current local sensitivities, integrating, as suggested by Strauss et al. (2005), best research evidence with clinical expertise and the patient's unique circumstances.

It was noted that the literature search did not retrieve studies reporting the rates of Gram-negative burn wound infection rates from the Centre for Disease Control in the United States. As reported by Wibbenmeyer et al. (2006), the Centre for Disease Control and Prevention (CDC) in Atlanta did not report burn wound infection rates but only pooled mean rates for device associated infection (CDC 2001), rendering this data ineligible for inclusion. This paucity of data is also acknowledges by leading experts in the field (Herndon 2009).

3.3 Risk Factors

Although risk factors leading to wound infection in the general adult civilian population have been extensively studied, it is clear from the literature that burn patients constitute a separate population (Dougherty and Waxman 1996; Santucci et al. 2003). Hence specific risk factors may be present in civilian adult burn patients that may govern the risk of Gram-negative BWI (Hodle et al. 2006; Weber and McManus 2004). These risk factors may relate to the specific pathophysiological changes following the burn trauma (such as TBSAB or burn depth), interventional procedures specific to burn patients such as shower hydrotherapy, or the different in-hospital length of stay typical of severely burnt patients. However, different methodologies and statistical techniques were used to investigate the potential associations and risk factors. A critical analysis and appraisal of the literature was therefore necessary to discern the methodological robustness underlying the validity of the reported results.

3.2.1 Total Body Surface Area, Burn Depth and Burn Injury Scores

Five narrative reviews investigated putative specific associations to BWI reported in the literature. Their results, synthesized in table 11, agreed about the association between BWI and TBSA. Mayhall et al. (2003) and Church et al. (2006) Edwards-Jones & Greenwood (2003) all provided level 5 evidence of this association, though well-conducted, referenced and argued narrative reviews, in agreement to Polavarapu et al.'s (2008) expert opinion article. These reviews reflected consensus in the literature only about a general link of TBSA to BWI. However given the possible biases characterising these studies, more robust literature was required to underpin recommendations.

Table 11: Risk Factors For Burn Wound Infection Identified from the Narrative Reviews

Paper	Risk Factors			
	TBSAB	LOS	Shower therapy*	Burn Depth
Mayhall (2000)	x	x	x	
Weber & McManus (2004)	x	x	x	x
Edwards-Jones& Greenwood (2003)	x			
Polavarapu (2008)	x			x
Church et al. (2006)	x			

TBSAB=total body surface area burnt; LOS=length of in-hospital stay; *(>30% mediates immunosuppressive effect); * Routine Communal Therapy.

Appelgren et al.'s (2002) study contained a second arm that investigated possible risk factors for BWI. They reported significant associations between BWI and TBSAB, burn injury scores, Length of Hospital Stay (LOS). These associations were reported through an analysis of putative risk variables between the infected (cohort) of patients and the matched non-infected cases (controls) moving forward in time, a methodology compatible to a prospective matched cohort study. Chi squared tests were used to investigate significant differences between the two groups over categorical risk variables. Their use was justified to compare categorical data sets. Assumptions including independence of observations, minimum sample sizes were plausibly met. The validity of this analysis would have been greater had random data sampling been used, to unequivocally justify the assumption of randomness. Yates' test was additionally used to prevent over-significance for small data samples. This increased the validity of the reported association at $p<0.001$. Appelgren et al.'s (2002) rigorous study design, which has already been appraised, indicated that this study's results were underpinned by level 2b evidence in Phillips et al. (2001). Furthermore Appelgren et al. (2002) observed that only 10 of 76 patients with BWI did not have full thickness injury. The association between full thickness burn and BWI from this study is therefore observational at best.

Table 12: Study Summary- Significant Associations Reported by the other Literature

Study	Evidence Level	Significant Association Reported			
		TBSAB	Burn severity Scores	Length of Stay	Burn Depth
Appelgren et al. (2002)	2b	X	x	x	
Wibbenmeyer et al. (2006)	2b	X			
Wong et al. (2002)	3b	X	x		X
Weber & McManus (2006)	4	X			
Ozkurt et al. (2005)				x	

Wibbenmeyer et al. (2006) also found a significant association between TBSA and incidence of nosocomial infection in burnt patients, supporting the findings of Appelgren et al. (2002). Wibbenmeyer et al. (2006) prospectively collected data from 157 burn patients' records over a one year period, and investigated BWI incidence rates (see Table 16) and risk factors for infection. This is the only reported study that, in the absence of universally accepted BWI diagnostic criteria, triangulated data from surgical and infection control personnel, increasing their methodological rigour. Furthermore, the control and sample groups' background characteristics were described in detail through the use of tabular data and chi squared tests, decreasing the risk of confounding factors. The statistical design was elegantly described, including the use of Wilcoxon's and Fisher tests to determine associations between putative risk factors and burn infection. The use of variance inflation factor to test for collinearity reduced the risk of highly correlated variables possibly explaining the same variability in the outcome hence being problematic during multivariate analysis (Dancey and Reidy 2004). Significant results in the univariate analyses were then forwarded to multiple logistic regression that reported a significant association of BWI incidence to TBSAB, and co-morbidities, and invasive device use. The tabulation of results and reporting P-values (p<0.05) increased the study's interpretability and rigour. Wibbenmeyer et al. (2006) also published odds ratios for TBSA as an independent risk factor for nosocomial infection. This enabled an interpretation of the size of magnitude of effect for this predictor. An OR of 1.2 (p<0.012) from data collected by burn surgeons and OR=1.21 (p<0.007) from data collected by infection control specialists reported a positive but weak predictive value.

42

Furthermore Wibbenmeyer et al.'s (2006) reported a two year study period which would eliminate the effects of seasonal variation that may have confounded the results of other studies such as Khorasani et al. (2008). The excellent methodological rigour, study/control definitions, and follow-up suggest that the evidence reported by Wibbenmeyer et al. (2006) regarding a significant association between nosocomial infection and TBSA is compatible with a robust prospective cohort trial (level 2b in Phillips et al. 2001), allowing extrapolation of the results to Gram-negative burn wound infection.

Weber and McManus' (2004 pp. A17) intended aims were 'to provide a comprehensive review'…..of the factors affecting risk of infection in burnt patients. Their paper actually focused on data retrieved from their own burn centre. Weber and McManus (2004) presented data retrieved from 645 patients over four years, to investigate the association between TBSA and BWI in their burn unit. This observational study suggested that a TBSA less than 30% was associated with a lower incidence of BWI than those over 30% (0.8% vs. 4.2% respectively).

The validity of Weber and McManus' (2004) results was limited by a number of considerations. The study sample was opportunistic rather than randomised, increasing possibility of selection bias. In contrast to Appelgren et al.'s (2002) rigorous design, basic demographic characteristics and background data were not reported or statistically analysed for lurking variables, increasing the possibility of confounding factors. Furthermore Weber and McManus (2004) reported that their study's duration was four years, but did not report individual patient follow-up. The evidence presented by Weber et al.'s (2004) would therefore only be compatible with level 4 in Phillips et al.'s (2001), hierarchy. Although their observational data was not found to be sufficiently robust that recommendations could be based on it independently, Weber and McManus (2004) provided further support to the findings of Wibbenmeyer et al. (2006) and Appelgren et al. (2002).

Data from Weber and McManus' (2004) own unit in Boston, USA was followed by a narrative review of the literature on risk factors for burn infection. This was the only narrative review to identify burn depth as a possible risk factor for burn wound infection, as well as shower hydrotherapy. The authors advocated the practice changes instituted at their own centre including individual shower and dressing change facilities. The organisation of this study suggested thoroughness of design. The time-limit for inclusion of studies (24 years) was reported. The review was logically organised and the principal literature was compared and synthesized. However, Weber and McManus (2004) did not report detailed inclusion criteria for the retrieved literature, which was not critically appraised. Furthermore, the literature review was used to justify practices in force at the authors' own burn centre suggesting the risk of clinical practice bias (Jadad 1998). These considerations suggested that evidence underpinning this part of Weber and McManus' (2004) study was comparable to level 5 in Phillips et al.'s (2001) hierarchy.

In order to determine risk factors for acquisition of Multidrug resistant Acinetobacter infection, Wong et al. (2002) performed a case-control study on 79 patients retrieved from over an 18 month period. Data from burn wounds and tracheal swabs performed every five days were obtained retrospectively from patient records. Their univariate analysis reported high TBSA, full thickness burns, intravascular lines, and increased admission APACHE (II) scores were associated with MR-Acinetobacter infection. Only increased admission APACHE (II) scores were reported by multivariate logistic regression to be a significant risk factor for acquisition of MR-Acinetobacter infection, although a numerical cut-off point for these increased scores was not reported.

A rigorous methodological design was reported to back these results. A detailed definition of inclusion criteria enabled clear characterisation of the cases (MR-Acinetobacter infected) and controls (other admissions). Furthermore, baseline characteristics were statistically tested using chi-squared for categorical variables and Mann-Whitney test for continuous variables, reducing the risk of confounding factors. The control group was exposed to identical inclusion and treatment criteria at the same hospital centre, further reducing the risk of confounding factors affecting validity. The authors unequivocally reported 'no omissions' in data collection. However, it would have been methodologically more robust to report a blind data collection to reduce the risk of retrieval bias. An identical validated and referenced microbiological analysis was also reported for both cases and controls decreasing the risk of measurement bias, while increasing reproducibility. Some methodological concerns may have affected the reported results' validity. Wong et al. (2002) specifically excluded patients surviving less than seven days. Intuitively, severely burnt patients would be less likely to survive with time. This could have skewed the results, possibly explaining why multiple logistic regression did not find TBSA to be a significant risk factor. The evidence presented by Wong et al. (2002) is therefore compatible with an individual case-control study with clearly defined case and control groups and adequate follow-up (Level 3b in Phillips et al.'s 2001 framework). One possible problem with applicability of this study is that the authors reported their association only with specific reference to Acinetobacter BWI. Wong et al. (2002) also pooled data from tracheal wounds to their BWI data. Their reported association therefore refers to a more general infection risk of Acinetobacter infection in burned patients. The methodological rigour however suggested that their results constituted level-3 evidence (Phillips et al, 2001) that could be extrapolated to Gram-negative burn wound infection providing further support to the findings of Appelgren et al. (2002).

3.2.2 Shower Therapy

Change from immersion to shower hydrotherapy has become a mainstay of contemporary burn wound treatment. However, the effects of shower hydrotherapy have recently become a source of dispute. Edwards-Jones & Greenwood (2003) and Polavarapu et al.'s (2008) narrative reviews both reported the fall in burn wound infections in the literature they synthesized. These assertions were contradicted by Mayhall (2003) and Church et al. (2006). The literature these two authors synthesized reported an unclear effect of this change in practice on burn wound infection rates. Additionally Church et al. (2006) synthesized outbreaks related to showering sprayers, plinths and boards. Conflicting evidence was therefore presented by level 5 studies relating to this important change in practice.

Simor et al. (2002) used multivariate logistic regression analysis to determine risk factors for Acinetobacter acquisition in a burns unit. Their case-control study included 29 cases with acquired Acinetobacter infection and 87 matched controls admitted within one month of the index cases, over a two year study period. Interestingly, hydrotherapy procedures were identified as an independent risk factor, even though it was explicitly reported that shower therapy only was used and not immersion. Various factors in the design of this study add credence to the reported results. Case and control characteristics were explicitly stated. Background characteristics were compared with chi squared tests reducing the risk of confounding factors. A 100% patient catchment rate was described for the study period, further decreasing the risk of selection bias. Furthermore the risk of selective patient loss was taken into account and mitigated by detailed follow-up, and justification of each patient that was excluded from the study based on the study's specific terms of reference, and validated operational definitions for BWI (Garner et al. 1988).

A meticulous stepwise methodology was reported both for the microbiological analysis of samples and for the statistical management of the collected data. Microbiological analysis was performed using validated and referenced techniques and triangulated with bacterial DNA testing. This rigorous approach ensured data for cases and controls was measured identically and increased internal validity. However, the lack of blinding in data collection and analysis may have introduced a degree of observer bias, which was mitigated to some extent by the rigorous approach described and the triangulation of microbiological and DNA results. A stepwise statistical approach was described increasing this study's reproducibility. Data was initially explored for risk factors using univariate analysis. Variables with a two-tailed $p<0.05$ were analysed with backward and forward stepwise logistic regression adjusted for potential confounding factors. Multiple logistic regression was appropriately applied to describe relationships between multiple possible risk factors and a dependent outcome variable.

The methodology of Simor et al. (2002) reflects a rigorous approach lending credence to their conclusions at level 3 evidence (Phillips et al. 2001). Immersion hydrotherapy was consigned to obsolescence due to reports linking it to increased infection rates and cross-contamination (Cardany et al. 1985; Church et al. 2006; Mayhall 2003). Hence identification of shower hydrotherapy as a risk for acquisition of Acinetobacter spp. infection with an Odds Ratio of 4.1 (P = 0.02) was a salient conclusion. This was corroborated by the finding of heavily contaminated surfaces used for shower therapy within the authors' institution reported within the discussion.

One particular issue with Simor et al.'s (2002) paper however is the conflict between data presented in tabular and text form. P values for TBSA, APACHE and FLAME scores were less than 0.05, however Simor et al. (2002) insist in their discussion that these factors 'did not appear to be associated with acquisition of multiresistant *A. baumannii'*. One possible explanation is the risk of multiple significance testing arising from using multiple univariate tests for significance (ex: Gosset/Chi squared/Fischer's tests) such that calculated p values may not be taken at face value.

Strauss et al. (2005) comment that relevance of the magnitude of the relative risk or odds ratio is also dependent on the validity of the underlying study design. Since the evidence supporting both risk factors has been shown by the critical appraisal to be of comparable robustness, it would appear that the magnitude of effect of shower hydrotherapy is greater than TBSAB as a predictor of burn infection.

The results of Simor et al. (2002) are in keeping with an observational study by Akin and Ozcan (2003) who used a disposable single-use sterilised plastic sheath to avoid burn wound cross-infection from shared shower facilities, then a problem in their institution. The change in practice was followed by weekly swabs from areas of the trolley for four years. This demonstrated a decrease in the rate of fomite colonization to zero.

Akin and Ozcan's (2003) design was in keeping with an unmatched cohort methodology. However this study did not measure exposure and outcome in the same, blinded objective fashion (Phillips et al. 2001). The recommendation presented by this study, is in keeping with level 4 evidence (Phillips et al. 2001). Applying a matched cohort methodology could have increased this study's interpretability by contrasting the results from an identical cohort sample taken from a trolley without the new modification. However, given that cross infection from shower facilities had already been identified as a potential risk factor, ethical considerations would not have allowed for this modification. It may thus be argued that Akin and Ozcan's (2003) design was the best possible methodology in the circumstances. Their simple and elegant proposition provided further support to Simor et al.'s (2002) identification of communal shower hydrotherapy facilities as an independent risk factor for burn wound infection.

3.2.3 Length of Stay

Ozkurt et al.'s (2005) retrospective cohort study reported length of in-hospital stay before isolation as a significant risk factor for acquiring resistant pseudomonas infection. Although the authors stated that 'a case-control study and a retrospective cohort study were conducted, these two study arms were not evident. An analysis of their study design actually reports a well defined cohort of patients was matched to a control sample and followed forward in time, in concordance to a retrospective cohort trial.

The study cohort was clearly defined through inclusion criteria, and the resulting patients admitted to the study were compared to their controls through chi squared tests, appropriately used for categorical variables, to test for significant differences. Through testing for known possible confounding factors, their risk was diminished. However, the introduction of blinding would have also decreased the risk of observer bias, increasing validity, as discussed in Simor et al. (2002). The validated referenced microbiological identification (API 20 NE system) and susceptibility tests (NCCSLS) described further increased reproducibility. Chi squared and Fisher tests were appropriately used to compare categorical data whereas Gosset's test and Mann-Whitney tests were used for parametrically and non-parametrically distributed continuous variables respectively. In concordance to Campbell (2001), multiple logistic regression was appropriately identified as the statistical method of choice to analyse the simultaneous effects of multiple categorical variables on a single variable. This increased the predictive value of Ozkurt et al.'s (2005) study. The rigorous design of Ozkurt et al.'s (2005) study in keeping with level 2b evidence (Phillips et al 2001).

Length of in-hospital stay before isolation was reported by Ozkurt et al. (2005) as being a risk factor for IRPA BWI, supporting the association between length of stay and Gram negative BWI reported by Appelgren et al (2002). Furthermore the authors report a 30% incidence of *Pseudomonas aeruginosa* in their unit, in keeping with the literature retrieved above. Interestingly however, TBSA was not associated to a significant risk of acquiring IRPA as opposed to ISPA. In fact Greenwood (2002) and Church et al. (2006) suggest that infection is a function of invasiveness which is determined by virulence factors, as opposed to antimicrobial resistance. The association between Length of Hospital Stay (LOS) and risk of infection is also supported by level five evidence from Mayhall (2000) and Weber & McManus (2004) as illustrated above.

Chim et al. (2007) and Appelgren et al. (2002) also investigated the relationship between infection and length of stay through the comparison of their sample of burned patients with BWI to a non-infected control burn group. Chim et al. (2007) appropriately used T-tests to test for association between nominal (infected vs. non-infected) and quantitative data (LOS). Appelgren et al. (2002) also found a significant association between median length of stay and burns infection. They also compared infected burn patients with a non-infected matched cohort group. Chi-squared tests with Yates' correction returned a significant association for burn infection and length of hospital stay in concordance to Chim et al. (2007). In-depth critical appraisal of Chim et al.'s (2007) methodology already returned a reliable and robust methodology compatible with level 3 evidence in Philips et al.'s (2001) hierarchy, while Appelgren et al.'s (2002) methodology was compatible with robust level 2b evidence. It may, therefore, be argued that the associations reported by these two authors were valid and supported by level 2b evidence (Appelgren et al. 2002) and level 3 evidence (2007). Although Chim et al. (2007) pooled data from BWI with other sources leading them to report on a more general association between infection in burnt hospitalised adult civilians, and length of stay, their methodological robustness and internal validity allowed confident extrapolation of the result to Gram-negative BWI as suggested by Phillips et al. (2001).Their results provide further support to associations between BWI and length of in-hospital stay before isolation reported by Ozkurt et al. (2005)

Chapter 4: Discussion

4.1 Introduction

In this study the formulation of clinical recommendations and suggestions for methodological advancement in future Gram negative burn wound research is based on a critical appraisal of the literature and judgement of the best currently available evidence. This study set out to investigate the aetiology incidence and specific risk factors of Gram-negative burn wound infection in hospitalised civilian adults. In this section the results of the literature synthesis will be summarised and discussed in line with the set purpose of the study.

4.2 Comparability of the literature

To investigate the aetiological profile and incidence of Gram-negative BWI in hospitalised adult civilians, it is essential to critically appraise current best evidence and standardise incidences regarding the definition of BWI.

Greenhalgh's (2007) criteria for defining BWI constitute current best evidence (see table 7). They took into account current clinical practice which increased their applicability to both bedside decision making and infection control reporting. Greenhalgh's (2007) definitions offer a good base for a common understanding of Gram-negative BWI which helps to increase diagnostic accuracy and reduce antibiotic over-prescribing. Several authors have underscored the need for an evidence-based approach in future definition to guide clinical decisions and comparability of research (see for example Appelgren et al. 2002; Church et al. 2006; Greenhalgh et al. 2007 Wibbenmeyer et al. 2006). Future research refining these criteria should therefore be evidence-based. Some of the different criteria used in the primary literature to define BWI are listed in table 13. This may pose problems for comparing primary studies. Greenhalgh et al.'s (2007) criteria could be generally adapted to validate BWI studies.

Table 13: Definitions of BWI Encountered in the Literature & Satisfaction of Criteria from Greenhalgh et al. (2007) by Working definitions in Primary Literature

Paper	Stated Actual Working Definitions from the Text	Criteria
Appelgren et al. (2002)	"Clinical and laboratory signs BWI are: (a) temperature >38.5 °C or <36 °C during at least 12 h or ongoing antipyretic therapy; (b) leukocyte count <4 or >12×109/l in blood (c) (c) C-reactive protein >50 mg/l" / 'burn wounds one swab from every 5% of burned surface' / a final decision was reached by consensus between the infectious disease consultant & burn surgeon	2c 1b
Chim et al. (2007)	'Signs and symptoms of infection commencing 48 h or more after admission to the Burns Centre were attributed to nosocomial infections Burn wound swabs sent every 5 days; Wound excisions sent for tissue histology	2b; 2c 1b 1c
Kaushik et al. (2001)	'Wound swabs were taken from the burn wounds and cultured';	1b
Khorasani et al. (2008)	"According to the clinical status of the participants, appropriate samples including wound swab, tissue biopsy […] were taken"	1b; 2a, 2b, 2c
(Komolafe et al. 2003);	"Specimens from burn injuries suspected to have been infected […] were analysed bacteriologically"	1A/B 2A/B/C
Lari and Alaghebandan (2000)	"Patients were swabbed on the 3rd and 7th day based on clinical judgment of infection. Infection and septicaemia were suspected when ... [list of signs]..."	1B & 2A/B/C
Ozumba et al. (2000)	Infection was diagnosed clinically. Clinical diagnosis guided surface wound swabbing when available.	2A/B/C +/-1B
Silla et al. (2006)	Working Definitions: 'Microbiology samples (wound swabs and blood cultures) were collected and processed routinely throughout according to clinical indication."	1A or 1B and 2A/B/ C
Singh et al. (2003)	"Wound swabs obtained from the burn patients were subjected to microbiological analysis". The isolates were identified by using standard microbiological techniques […] Any repeat sample or isolate obtained on more than one occasion from the same patient was not included in the study.	1B

NI= nosocomial infection

Similarly standardisation of incidence rates for Gram-negative BWI was essential to ensure that the synthesis and final recommendations of this study were based on a valid comparison of the primary literature. However the process also served to inform a knowledge gap that had not been attempted in earlier reviews (Church et al. 2006; Edwards-Jones and Greenwood 2003; Mayhall 2003) and facilitated a clearer reflection on Gram-negative BWI incidences in hospitalised civilian adults.

Whilst Greenhalgh et al.'s (2007) diagnostic criteria for burn wound infection are being recommended as operational definitions for future research clinical bedside use and infection surveillance future diagnostic criteria need to be evidence-based. To facilitate comparison, standardised incidence rates should be used.

4.3 Aetiology and Incidence of Gram-Negative Burn Wound Infection in Hospitalised Adult Civilians

The critical appraisal process elucidated a similar Gram-negative bacteriological profile from the primary literature despite varying study methodologies, samples, durations and distinct geographic settings. *Pseudomonas aeruginosa, Acinetobacter, Klebsiella, Enterobacter, E.coli* and *Proteus* were consistently reported as the commonest causes of BWI in hospitalised adult civilians, with the apparent exception of *E. coli* (Appelgren et al. 2002; Silla et al. 2006), and *Acinetobacter* (Khorasani et al. 2008). Table 14 illustrates that this finding is supported by a body of evidence consisting of 16 studies: 4 robust studies at level two supported by 2 level-three studies and 5 at level-four within Phillips et al.'s (2001) hierarchy.

	Paper	Level	Salient Conclusions
Narrative Reviews	Edwards-Jones & Greenwood (2003) Church et al. (2006) Mayhall (2003) Polavarapu (2008)	5+ 5	*Pseudomonas aeruginosa* reported as commonest Gram-negative BWI aetiology. Synthesis on other Gram-negative aetiologies of BWI was absent, creating a gap in the literature. The literature suggested expert opinion to concur that different burn centres are bacteriologically distinct
Cohort Studies	Chim et al. (2007)	3	*Pseudomonas aeruginosa; Acinetobacter baumannii; Klebsiella pneumoniae; E. coli; Enterobacter* spp. and *Proteus* spp. commonest BWI. Blast patients exhibited increased rates of Acinetobacter infection.
	Appelgren et al. (2002)	2b	-*Pseudomonas aeruginosa; Acinetobacter baumannii; Klebsiella pneumoniae; Enterobacter* spp. and *Proteus* spp. commonest BWI. -*E. coli* not reported as a significant pathogen. -BWI defined in concordance between surgeons and ICS teams
	Wibbenmeyer et al.	2b	*Pseudomonas aeruginosa* commonest Gram-ve BWI Different operational definitions may result in misreporting of data and over-prescription of antibiotics
	Khorasani et al. (2008)	2b	*Pseudomonas aeruginosa* commonest pathogen; Acinetobacter not reported as significant BWI. Citrobacter outbreak reported.
	Lari & Alaghebandan (2000)	3	Primary BWI over first week: *Pseudomonas* spp. *Acinetobacter; Enterobacter* spp. NO data on *Klebsiella* spp.; *E. coli; Proteus* spp.
	Agnihotri et al. (2004a) Kaushik et al. (2001)	4 4-	*Pseudomonas aeruginosa; Acinetobacter baumannii; Klebsiella pneumoniae; Enterobacter* spp. and *Proteus* spp. commonest BWI. No data on *E. coli*
	Ozumba et al. (2000) Komolafe et al. (2003)	4 4-	*Pseudomonas aeruginosa; Acinetobacter baumannii; Klebsiella pneumoniae; Enterobacter* and Proteus commonest BWI Profiling may be the only indication of BWI aetiology when no microbiology is available due to cost
Case-ctrl	Singh et al. (2003)	4	*Pseudomonas aeruginosa; Acinetobacter baumannii; Klebsiella pneumoniae; E. coli* and *Proteus* spp. commonest BWI. No data on *Enterobacter*. Routine bacterial profiling helps antibiotic prescribing & reduces resistance
Audit	Silla et al. (2006)	2	*Pseudomonas* spp. & *Acinetobacter* spp. reported as commonest primary BWI. Significant differences between 'routine' admissions and Bali-Blast victims due to delayed transfer, co-trauma, and increased TBSA

The apparent discrepancies reported by Khorasani et al. (2008) with respect to *Acinetobacter* and Appelgren et al. (2002) Silla et al. (2006), regarding *E. coli* (table 15) may be challenged through three possible lurking variables identified in the critical analysis. Rather than truly distinct bacteriological profiles, the critical appraisal process suggested that seasonal variation (Gales et al. 2001; McDonald et al. 1999; Perencevich et al. 2008) may have affected Khorasani et al. (2008) results. Furthermore a decreased accuracy of identification of *Acinetobacter* as a significant pathogen in local laboratories (Abbassi et al. 2006) could have possibly acted as a confounding factor, one hitherto un-identified by the literature. Similarly, the absence of *E. coli* from Appelgren et al.'s (2002) study can be attributed to their stringent patient-hygiene and infection control institutional policy. In fact the only other study not to report *E. coli* among the causes of primary incidence of Gram-negative BWI was Silla et al. (2006), where similar extensive patient hygiene and general infection control practices were described.

Table 15: Common Gram-Negative BWI Bacteriological Profile Identified in the Primary Literature, Exception and probable Lurking Variable

Gram Negative BWI	Exception	Probable Reason from Critical Appraisal
Pseudomonas aeruginosa	NA	
Acinetobacter spp.	Khorasani et al. (2008)	Seasonal variation; Specific Low Diagnostic Lab Accuracy for Acinetobacter
Klebsiella spp.	NA	
E. coli	Appelgren et al. (2002) Silla et al. (2006)	*E. coli* associated to faecal contamination. Specific practices to prevent in place at both study centres
Enterobacter spp.	NA	
Proteus spp.	NA	

A common BWI Gram-negative bacteriological profile in hospitalised civilian adults informed the purpose of this study through providing robust evidence for the choice of initial antimicrobial therapy from diagnosis to the arrival of the final microbiology report. Based on the current best evidence, this initial antimicrobial therapy should cover for Pseudomonas, Klebsiella, Acinetobacter, *E. coli, Enterobacter*, and *Proteus* integrated to the local susceptibilities. This result challenges conclusions of previous single studies that burn centres are bacteriologically different (Agnihotri et al. 2004; Edwards-Jones and Greenwood 2003;

Kaushik et al. 2001), and provides credence for transferability of research findings between different burns units. Having established that the evidence suggests a common Gram-negative BWI bacteriological profile in the primary literature regarding hospitalised civilian adults, the next step is a consideration of whether current best evidence also suggests a similarity in the incidence rates.

4.3.1 Incidence of Gram-Negative Burn Wound Infection in Hospitalised Adult Civilians

The incidence rates of Gram-negative BWI in hospitalised civilian adults based on current best evidence suggest a mean incidence rate of 156 Gram-negative BWI/1000 patient-years in hospitalised civilian adults. Unstandardised raw data (Figure 1) suggests that the majority of BWI in hospitalised civilian adults is caused by Gram-negative infection (mean 64.1%).

We explored this observation through providing standardized incidence rates for each of the commonest Gram-negative BWI in hospitalised civilian adults from the retrieved primary literature (table 16). It contrasts with the incomplete syntheses presented by earlier reviews (Church et al. 2006; Edwards-Jones and Greenwood 2003) which only identified pseudomonal infection as the commonest Gram-negative BWI in this patient group.

Percentage of BWI infection Caused by Gram-Negative BWI

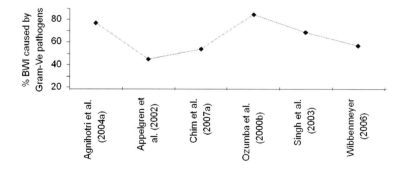

Figure 1: Percentage of Burn Wound Infections Caused by Gram-Negative Pathogens

Data-distribution of the standardised incidence rates for each pathogen in the identified Gram-negative BWI profile is represented by a box-whisker plot (Figure 5). Although further statistical analysis was not possible due to heterogeneous methodologies of the primary studies, a descriptive analysis of data-distribution strongly suggests a limited dispersion of data from the mean with little variation between the first and third quartile, or even between outliers (indicated by whiskers) than may be intuitively expected if each individual centre had a completely unique bacteriological profile. *Pseudomonas aeruginosa* was reported as the most incident Gram-negative BWI, followed by *Klebsiella, Acinetobacter, Enterobacter Proteus* and *E. coli*, with their respective mean incidence rates synthesised in table 17. As Silla et al. (2006) and Lari and Alaghebandan's (2000) studies investigated primary incidence and incidence over post-burn week 1 respectively, they could not be synthesized with the rest of the data in Figure .

Table 16: Incidence of Burn Wound Infection in Hospitalised Civilian Adults
(Incidence Rates Expressed in terms of New Cases per 1000 patients per year)

Study and Evidence Level (Phillips et al. 2001)	Patients (n)	Study Duration (Years)	BWI Incidence	Gram-ve BWI incidence	Pseudomonas Aeruginosa	Acinetobacter	Enterobacter	Klebsiella	E. coli	Proteus	Mixed Infection (%)
Agnihotri et al. (2004)	4	692	5	192	148	111	13.8	7.5	7.5	ND	6.2	13%
Appelgren et al. (2002)	2b	230	3	155	70	39	4.3	14	11.5	0	ND	12%
Chim et al. (2007)	3	57	5	163	89	31.4	38.4	21	14	3.5	3.5	ND
Khorasani (2008)	2b	113	0.5	530	ND	265	ND	ND	ND	ND	ND	ND
Ozumba & Jiburum (2000)	4	71	5	253	174	39.4	ND	30.8	67.6	11	25.2	6.1%
Singh et al. (2003)	4	759	5	151	86.2	46	13.4	ND	50	5.6	10.4	40%
Wibben-meyer et al. (2006)	2b	157	1	382	ND	152	ND	ND	ND	ND	ND	ND
Silla et al. (2006)*	2b	59	0.25	59	ND	200	200	80	80	ND	ND	ND
Lari and Alagheband an (2000) *	3b	582	2.5	438	370	128	38	10	ND	ND	ND	ND

Average rate of Gram-negative BWI 156 (hospitalised civilian adults)

Percentage of BWI in hospitalised civilian adults due to the identified bacteriological profile = 64.1%)

* These studies investigated *primary* incidence of Gr-ve BWI. As their standardised incidence ratios could not be confidently compared to the rest of the literature they were not included in fig. 2

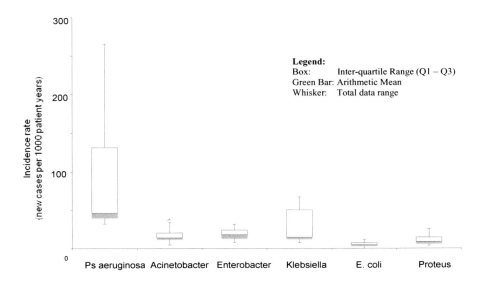

Figure 2: Box-Plot Graph for Incidence Rates of Gram-Negative BWI In Hospitalised Civilian Adults

---

Table 17: Data Synthesis From Figure 2

	Pseudomonas	Klebsiella	Acinetobacter	Enterobacter	Proteus	E .coli
Mean	97.6	30.2	17.4	18.2	4	5

Lari and Alaghebandan (2000) and Silla et al. (2006) investigated primary incidence over 1 week, hence could not be included in Figure 5.

The box-whisker plot for pseudomonas exhibits the widest dispersion of data. This may be explained by the fact that crude infection incidence rates may vary depending on general infection control variation between burn units. If the incidence rates of pseudomonas are standardised as a quotient of the total BWI rates at individual burn centres, Figure 3 suggests that the standardised incidence rates in 8 randomly selected centres are actually similar.

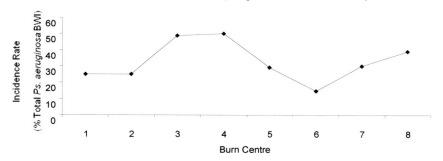

**Incidence Rate of Pseudomonas aeruginosa BWI as Quotient of
Total BWI in Each Burn Centre (Hospitalized Civilian Adults)**

Figure 3: Incidence Rates of Pseudomonas aeruginosa BWI as Quotient of Total BWI
In 8 Burn Centres (Hospitalised Civilian Adults)

Due to internal validity problems inherent in Kaushik et al. (2001) and Komolafe et al. (2003) level 4 - (Phillips et al. 2001), these were excluded from the formulation of incidence rates. However Komolafe et al.'s (2003) paper was a still a valuable contribution to this study because, in concordance to Ozumba and Jiburum (2000) it enabled a reflection on the clinical relevance of this study's recommendations to institutions regularly facing financial challenges to best practice, where microbiology results may not be available once throughout the course of Gram-negative BWI. This scenario provides further scope and clinical value for this study's final recommendations.

Complementing these studies, Silla et al. (2006) provided level 2b evidence (Phillips et al. 2001) that BWI rates were significantly increased and Acinetobacter was significantly more common in their cohort from the Bali terrorist attacks. Chim et al. (2007), the only other study with similar findings actually admitted patients from the Jakarta-Marriot terrorist event. Robust evidence at levels 2b and 3 in Phillips et al.'s (2001) hierarchy therefore suggests that Acinetobacter infection may be more incident and should be suspected in this patient group. It may therefore be argued that this difference in Silla et al. (2006) and Chim et al.'s (2007) results is due to the fact that patients from terror attacks could represent a different sub-population and were subject to lurking variables that would not be expected in hospitalised civilian adults.

Five studies reported on the incidence of mixed infections. Their studies provided level 2b evidence (Appelgren et al. 2002; Silla et al. 2006) supported by level 4 evidence (Ozumba and Jiburum 2000) that the majority of reported infections were mono-microbial. Although mixed organisms were reported to cause a minority of BWI, their incidence was not negligible (range 6.1% to 40%). The wider literature suggests that this finding may be clinically significant since intra-and inter-species mixed infections may have a major impact in the development of clinical infection. This could be possibly due to induced gene expression (Church et al. 2006) co-expression of virulence factors (Edwards-Jones and Greenwood 2003), and the risk of polymicrobial bacteraemia which is significantly associated to an increased risk of mortality (Appelgren et al. 2002).

Current best evidence thus strongly suggests similarity in the Gram-negative BWI profiles: *Pseudomonas aeruginosa*, *Acinetobacter* spp., *Enterobacter* spp., *E. coli*, and *Proteus* spp. are the commonest causes of Gram-negative BWI in hospitalised civilian adults. Appraisal analysis and synthesis of the evidence also suggests that the standardised incidence rates of this microbial profile may be similar across the burn centres studied. It may therefore be argued that the choice of the 'best guess' initial antimicrobial therapy from diagnosis to arrival of the final microbiology report should cover for *Pseudomonas aeruginosa*, *Klebsiella* spp., *Acinetobacter* spp., *Enterobacter* spp., *Proteus* spp. and *E. coli*, integrated to the local susceptibilities present at a particular burns centre. This is supported by 4 level-two studies, 2 studies at level three and 5 studies at level four in Phillips et al.'s (2001) hierarchy. These findings also challenge earlier studies which asserted a unique bacteriological profile for each individual burn centre. Furthermore, identification of this Gram-negative bacteriological profile as the commonest cause of BWI from the synthesized literature underscores their clinical relevance despite not being as well publicised as MRSA in both peer reviewed (McConnel 2006) and lay literature (BBC 2009) and may also help argue the case for resource-allocation to development of new antimicrobial agents. Robust level 2b and 3 evidence (Phillips et al. 2001) also suggests a low threshold of suspicion for Acinetobacter BWI in patients with a history of being involved in terrorist events.

4.4 Specific Risk Factors for Gram-negative BWI in Hospitalised Adult Civilians

Shower therapy, burn depth, TBSA, burn injury scores, length of hospital stay were investigated by 11 primary studies as possible risk factors for Gram-negative burn wound infection in hospitalised civilian adults (table 18).

Table 18: Literature Synthesis Regarding
TBSA; Depth of Burn, and Burn Severity Scores As possible risk factors for BWI
(X= significant Association reported)

Study & Level of Evidence underpinning Results (Phillips et al. 2001)		TBSAB	Burn injury Scores	LOS	Shower therapy**	Burn Depth
			Risk Factors Investigated			
Mayhall (2000)		x		x	x	
Weber & McManus (2004)		x*		x	x	x
Edwards-Jones & Greenwood (2003)	5	x*				
Polavarapu (2008)		x				x
Church et al. (2006)		x			x	
Appelgren et al. (2002)	2b	x	x	x		
Ozkurt et al. (2005)	2b			x		
Simor et al. (2002)	2b				x	
Weber (2004)	4	x				
Wibbenmeyer et al. (1993)	2b	x				
Wong (2002)	3b	x	x	x		x

NI= Not investigated by the primary study; LOS = length of in-hospital stay; TBSAB= Total Body Surface Area Burnt

61

4.4.1 Total Body Surface Area

Evidence about the association and predictive significance of TBSA and incidence of Gram-negative BWI was conflicting. At univariate analysis level both Appelgren et al. (2002) and Wibbenmeyer et al. (2006) reported a significant association between TBSA and incidence of burn infection with $p<0.05$ level of significance, providing robust evidence at level 2b and 3 in Philips et al.'s (2001) hierarchy to substantiate this association. Further support for this relationship was provided by expert opinion (Church et al. 2006; Edwards-Jones and Greenwood 2003; Mayhall 2003; Polavarapu et al. 2008). At multivariate analysis level, however, Wong et al.'s (2002) conclusion that TBSA was not a significant predictor of multiresistant Acinetobacter burn infection (level 3b) challenged Wibbenmeyer et al. (2006) who maintained that TBSA was a significant predictor of infection in burn patients, including Gram-negative BWI, (Odds Ratio of 1.21 at $p<0.05$, level 2b evidence). This apparent conflict may be explained in terms of disparate rigour in the logistic regression approach, possible data contamination and methodological rigour. Wibbenmeyer et al.'s (2006) structured approach to logistic regression, avoided the pitfalls of unexplored data collinearity (Armitage et al. 2002) present in Wong et al. (2002). Wong et al. (2002) also pooled a minority of samples from tracheal wound swabs to the BWI data, possibly leading to data contamination.

On balance current best evidence, therefore, suggests a significant association between TBSAB, and increased Gram-negative BWI incidence. Further support to this association was provided by Weber and McManus'(2004) level four study (Phillips et al. 2001) who observed a higher BWI incidence in patients with more than 30% TBSA. It may also be argued that though TBSA was a significant predictor of burn infection, an odds ratio of 1.21 suggests that the magnitude of effect for this predictor is weak. The robustness of the studies underpinning this evidence allowed confident extrapolation to the risk of acquiring Gram-negative BWI.

4.4.2 Burn Depth & Severity of Burn Injury

The literature reviewed by Weber and McManus (2004) and Polavarapu (2008) suggested that the presence of full thickness burns may increase burn wound infection rates. Appelgren et al. (2002) furthered this insight through a descriptive exploration of their data, suggesting a link between the presence of full thickness burns and increased incidence of BWI. In contrast Wong et al. (2002) used univariate analysis to provided level 3b evidence that the presence of full thickness skin burn is statistically associated to the risk of multiresistant *Acinetobacter* spp. BWI, albeit at a significance value of p<0.10.

Although current best evidence does suggest a link between the presence of FTSB and increased incidence of BWI, it could therefore be argued that the evidence is presently weak. A possible explanation could be that current best evidence investigated the association between presence, rather than the extent of FTSB, and incidence of BWI. Furthermore, during early excision and grafting both partial and full thickness wounds are converted to surgical wound and grafted. Intuitively, converting both types of wounds into a surgical wound may account for this disparity in the results.

Both Appelgren et al. (2002) and Wong et al. (2002) argued that scores denoting severity of burn injury were associated to an increased risk of infection in hospitalised civilian adults. On a univariate analysis level, ABSI scores (Appelgren et al. 2002) and increased admission APACHE (II) (Wong et al. 2002) scores were both significantly associated to infection in burn patients (p<0.05). These results were supported by robust level 2 and 3B evidence. The rigour of these studies' methodology allowed for confident extrapolation to the incidence of Gram-negative BWI for the purposes of underscoring recommendations as advised by Phillips et al.'s (2001) hierarchy of evidence tools. Although on a multivariate logistic regression level Wong et al. (2002) found that increased admission APACHE (II) scores were significantly predicative of multiresistant Acinetobacter infection in burn patients, the magnitude of effect of this predictor was weak (RR=1.33). Furthermore, the problems with their multivariate logistic regression methodology suggested that this factor should be viewed as a robust association rather than a weak predictor in the formulation of recommendations. It is being argued that level 2b and 3b evidence exists to suggest that scores denoting severity of injury may be significantly associated with an increased incidence of infection in burnt patients. However, the evidence underscoring an increased admission APACHE (II) score as a significant predictor of Gram-negative BWI is weak and further robust studies are required to substantiate this predictor.

Current best evidence therefore supports a significant association between TBSA, ABSI scores and admission APACHE (II) and increased incidence of Gram-negative infection. Level 2b evidence also suggests that TBSA is predictor of Gram-negative BWI but the magnitude of this association is weak. On the other hand, the evidence supporting an association between burn depth and increased incidence of Gram-negative BWI is weak, and could not be confidently used to formulate recommendations. These conclusions may form a rationale for recommending a higher index of suspicion where the burn patient's history suggests the presence of these associations. Where access to resources that reduce risk of infection is limited, the presence of these associations may form an evidence-basis for apportioning these resources between patients. Identification of these associations, the strength of the evidence with which they are supported, and the strength of association on univariate and multivariate analysis may direct future studies investigating statistical models of Gram –negative burn wound infection risk in hospitalised civilian adults.

4.4.3 Shower therapy

Simor et al. (2002) reported that shower hydrotherapy was a significant predictive risk factor for the acquisition of *Acinetobacter baumannii* burn wound infection. Their robust, well-designed case-control study provided level 3 evidence that procedures preformed in the shower therapy room carried an Odds Ratio (OR) of 4.1 (p=0.02) of developing multiresistant *Acinetobacter baumannii*. BWI. Validity of odds ratios is a function of both the strength of the underlying evidence and the OR magnitude (Strauss et al. 2005). A critical appraisal of this study strongly suggested that it is sufficiently robust, and that the OR magnitude of 4.1 was significantly high, to infer a strong association between procedures in the hydrotherapy room and risk of Acinetobacter BWI. Weber and McManus (2004) provided further level 4 support to this association.

Possible solutions to this significant predictor were proposed by Weber and McManus (2004) whose level 4 evidence (Phillips et al. 2001) advised that patients at increased risk of infection, including those with higher TBSA and burn depth, should avoid procedures in shower therapy rooms. Akin and Oscan's (2003) elegant and simple conclusion that disposable ethylene sheets may significantly decrease cross-infection rates during shower therapy is also identified as a feasible and cheap solution to counter this problem. It is surprising that despite the significance of Simor et al.'s (2002) findings few studies have investigated possible solutions to this significant risk which should have stimulated higher research interest.

The evidence provided by Weber and McManus (2004) Simor et al. (2002) and Akin and Oscan's (2003) studies suggest that shower therapy is a significant predictor of Gram-negative BWI in hospitalised civilian adults. It may be argued that this evidence forms a rationale against common shower therapy facilities. When their use is deemed necessary, disposable sterilised plastic sheets should be used to isolate patients form fomite contact. Dissemination of information should be directed to nursing staff, to maximise the impact that this simple but feasible and effective recommendation would have on Gram-negative BWI hospitalised civilian adults.

4.4.4 Length of Hospital Stay

The reviewed literature reported consensus on the association between length of in-hospital stay and incidence of Gram-negative BWI. The principal study supporting this association was carried out by Ozkurt et al.'s (2005) who provided robust evidence, that length of in-hospital stay before isolation is significantly associated to Imipenem-Resistant *Pseudomonas aeruginosa*. Furthermore, their conclusion that LOS is a predictor for IR-Pseudomonas BWI is statistically significant and has an increased magnitude of effect (OR of 3.1) supported by a robust level-two methodology enabling these conclusions to be confidently applied to the final recommendations. Appelgren et al. (2002) and Chim et al. (2007) also provided consistent evidence of a significant association between LOS and incidence of BWI. This level 2b and 3 evidence was concordant to the narrative reviews of Mayhall (2000) and & McManus (2004) who argued for this association based on a narrative synthesis of their retrieved literature. However these studies investigated the association of LOS to burns infections in general. While their robust methodology confidently allowed extrapolation of their conclusions to Gram-negative BWI, this could only be used to provide more support to

Ozkurt et al. (2005) rather than independently underpin evidence-based recommendations.

It may, therefore, be argued that length of in-hospital stay before isolation is significantly associated to risk of acquiring BWI. Based on current best evidence this period should be kept to a minimum whenever possible. At the same time it is recognised that pressures on isolation room demand are a ubiquitous challenge in hospitals. In case of limited availability, priority should be afforded to patients with higher TBSA, increased APACHE (II) and ABSI scores since these patients are more susceptible to infection.

Current best evidence reported odds ratios on three significant predictive factors for increased incidence of Gram-negative BWI in hospitalised civilian adults. Simor et al.'s (2002) study stated an OR of 4.1 (p<0.02) for procedures in common shower therapy rooms; Wibbenmeyer et al.'s (2006) study reported an OR of 1.21 (p<0.05) for TBSA and Ozkurt et al.'s (2005) study established an OR of 3.1 (p<0.0012) for length of stay before isolation. An appraisal of these magnitudes of effect as suggested by Strauss et al. (2005), surprisingly suggests that TBSA is less significant a predictor than LOS or procedures in a common shower therapy ambient. Given the reason for wholesale change from immersion to shower therapy, these results highlight an urgent need to minimise procedural risk associated to shower hydrotherapy, and educate nursing staff.

4.5 Suggestions for Refining Current Methodological Designs

The aetiology incidences and risk factors for Gram-negative BWI in hospitalised civilian adults remain under-studied, despite their importance. Appelgren et al.'s (2002) study was the only reported European attempt to continuously update the burn surgeon with evidence regarding Gram-negative BWI profiles, on which to base clinical decisions. The CDC (USA) currently does not report data on BWI (Gallagher 2009; Herndon 2009 personal communication). A critical analysis of the reviewed studies revealed common features consistent with robust methodological design, but also some consistent concerns to internal validity which should be addressed in future studies. An increase in robust publications would broaden the limited amount of current best evidence on which this study was based.

Although RCT's would be methodologically ideal to study aetiology intentional exposure to harmful pathogens would be clearly unethical (Crombie 2008). Therefore, a prospective cohort design may be better suited towards this purpose. This study design would reduce the potential retrieval and ascertainment bias that reduced rigour and validity of retrospective designs such as Kaushik et al. (2001). Integration of evidence from an on-going prospective cohort study integrated to a web-based platform such as that used by the British Association of Antimicrobial Chemotherapy website (BSAC 2009) would provide an ideal method for dissemination of up-to-date evidence for burn clinicians.

A comprehensive précis illustrating the state of predating literature, its completeness and validity would assist the reader in identifying clearly the problems under investigation identify the literature gap addressed and avoid un-necessary duplication, as occurred to Kaushik et al. (2001). A general awareness and common application of BWI diagnostic criteria, such as Greenhalgh et al.'s (2007) would also help in establishing acceptable definitions that would enhance comparability of results between different burn centres and enhance transference of research findings. Also, reportage of incidence rates in a standardised format (Jewell 2004) would enable comparability between studies.

More rigourous designs and sampling techniques and statistical rigour need to be applied in future BWI studies Opportunistic sampling, with the inherent risk of sample bias and lurking variables was a concern with some studies (example: Komolafe et al. (2003), and Kaushik et al. (2001). Randomised inclusion of patients (Jadad 1998) would reduce the threats to validity resulting from opportunistic sampling. A calculation of sample-size and power would increase the applicability of these studies to the general population of hospitalised civilian adults admitted to the institution over a defined period of time. Furthermore, more studies that focus on matched cohort groups would improve identification of risk factors for Gram-negative BWI (see Appelgren et al. 2002).

Literature regarding transport and culture media used is scarce (Agnihotri et al. 2004; Khorasani et al. 2008): its standardisation would reduce the possibility of it acting as a confounding factor. Furthermore, a description of validated microbial identification methods should be complemented by reporting the performance of the participating laboratories against reference centres, minimising lurking factors external to the study, illustrated by the challenge Abbasi et al.'s (2006) findings presented to Kaushik et al. (2001).

The use of computerised data entry (example Appelgren et al. 2002) facilitates data collection and mitigates the risk of retrieval bias. Blinded data collection would reduce the risk of observer and retrieval bias. Inclusion of new data only in case of clinically-significant pathogen changes, such as reported by Agnihotri et al. (2004) would reduce data duplication risks. Follow-up until discharge or death as illustrated by Appelgren et al. (2002) would satisfy adequacy of follow-up and identify sample attrition increasing study rigour. Furthermore, a time-span of five years such as reported by Singh et al. (2003) and Chim et al. (2007) would reduce the risk of seasonal variation that may have confounded Khorasani et al.'s (2008) results. Finally, the use of model diagnostics in studies investigating risk and predictors of increased Gram-negative BWI could improve the predictive power of antecedents.

Chapter 5: Recommendations, Implications for Practice & Conclusions

The evidence-based approach adopted in this study allowed an in-depth appraisal of the primary studies for rigour, robustness validity and impact, in order to determine the aetiological profile incidence and specific risk-factors for Gram-negative BWI in hospitalised civilian adults. This approach therefore added to the knowledge base by providing evidence-based recommendations for clinical practice and future research in the initial management of Gram-negative BWI in hospitalised civilian adults with a robust and valid foundation. It is intended that conscientious and judicious use of these recommendations would support clinical expertise in individual patient scenarios and local susceptibility profiles. These recommendations are summarised in table 19.

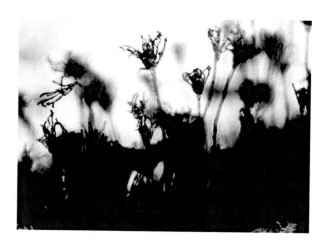

Figure 4: Penicillium culture. Evidence-based treatment is paramount in the post-penicillin era (Weinbren 2009)

Table 19: Evidence-Based Recommendations for Clinical Practice

Recommendation 1:   (Grade B)

Based on the current best evidence, the initial antimicrobial therapy from diagnosis to arrival of the final microbiology report should cover for *Pseudomonas aeruginosa*, *Klebsiella* spp, *Acinetobacter* spp., *E. coli*, *Enterobacter* spp, *Proteus* spp. integrated to the local susceptibilities.

Supporting Studies (Level of Evidence after Phillips et al. 2001

Appelgren et al. (2002) [level 2b]   Wibbenmeyer et al. (2006)   [level2b]   Khorasani et al. (2008) [level2b]
Chim et al. (2007)   [level 3]   Lari & Alaghebandan (2000) [level 3]
Agnihotri et al. (2004) [level 4]   Ozumba and Jiburum (2000) [level 4]   Singh et al. (2003)   [level 4]

Recommendation 2:   (Grade B)

Current best evidence suggests that the incidence of Gram-negative BWI is significantly increased in blast injury victims (such as civilian victims of terror attacks), with a significantly increased incidence of *Acinetobacter* spp. BWI. Initial antimicrobial therapy should therefore cover for *Acinetobacter* BWI.

Supporting Evidence & Level (Phillips et al. 2001)
Silla et al. (2006) [Level 2b]   Chim et al. (Chim et al. 2007) [Level 3b]

Recommendation 3:   (Grade C)

It is recommended that High TBSA; increased ABSI; Admission APACHE (II) scores; communal shower therapy; LOS should be included as exploratory variables in the investigation of logistic regression model building for predictors of Gram-negative BWI in hospitalised civilian adults.

Supporting Evidence & Level (Phillips et al. 2001)
Appelgren et al.'s (2002) [Level 2b*] Wibbenmeyer et al.'s (2006) [Level 2b*]
Weber and McManus (2004) [Level 4] Polavarapu (2008) [level 5]
Mayhall (2003) [level 5] Edwards-Jones & Greenwood (2003) [level 5] Church et al. (2006) [level 5]

Recommendation 4:   (Grade C)

The presence of high TBSA; increased ABSI; increased APACHE (II) scores; and increased LOS warrant a high index of suspicion for development of Gram-negative BWI should be included in the risk assessment process for patients developing Gram-negative BWI. Where access to resources that reduce risk of infection is limited, the presence of these associations forms evidence-bases for apportioning these resources between patients.

Supporting Evidence & Level (Phillips et al. 2001)

Appelgren et al.'s (2002) [Level 2b*] Wibbenmeyer et al.'s (2006) [Level 2b*]
Weber and McManus (2004) [Level 4] Polavarapu (2008) [level 5]
Mayhall (2003) [level 5] Edwards-Jones & Greenwood (2003) [level 5] Church et al. (2006) [level 5]

Recommendation 5: (Grade C)

Procedures in common shower therapy facilities should be avoided in favour of individual facilities. When necessary, sterilised disposable plastic sheets should be used to isolate patients from fomite contact.

Supporting Evidence & Level (Phillips et al. 2001)
Simor et al. (2002) [Level 2b*]   Akin & Ozcan (2003) [Level 4]   Weber & Mc Manus (2004) [Level 4]
Weber and McManus (2004) [Level 5]; Mayhall (2003) [level 5];   Church et al. (2006) [level 5]

Recommendation 6: (Grade C)

It is recommended that future studies clarify the role of burn depth to incidence of Gram-negative BWI. Current best evidence favours the possibility of this association, but the strength of the current best evidence is not sufficient to underscore recommendations.

Supporting Studies (Level of Evidence after Phillips et al. 2001)
Weber and McManus (2004) Polavarapu's (2008) and Appelgren et al. (2002)

Recommendation 7: (Grade B)

Greenhalgh et al.'s (2007) diagnostic criteria for burn wound infection are recommended as operational definitions for future studies; clinical bedside use and infection surveillance, as they constitute current best evidence.

Supporting Studies (Level of Evidence after Phillips et al. 2001)

Appelgren et al. (2002)   [Level 2b]   Wibbenmeyer et al. (2006) [level 2b]
Greenhalgh et al. (2007)   [level 5]   Church et al. (2006)   [level 5]

Current best evidence strongly suggests that *Pseudomonas aeruginosa*, *Klebsiella* spp., *Acinetobacter* spp., *Enterobacter* spp., *E. coli* and *Proteus* spp. are the commonest causes of Gram-negative burn wound infection in hospitalised civilian adults. It also suggests that the standardised incidence rates of this bacteriological profile may be similar across the primary literature. Apparent differences in the primary literature may be due to methodological differences between studies rather than unique institutional microbiological profiles. Application of this finding, coupled to local expertise on the individual patient circumstances and local sensitivity profiles should therefore inform the choice of initial 'best guess' antimicrobial therapy, during the time period from diagnosis of Gram-negative infection, to arrival of the final microbiology report. This would be in communion with Sackett and Rosenberg's principle of conscientious and judicious use of current best evidence applied to individual patient circumstances. These Grade B recommendations were underscored by robust level 2 evidence (Appelgren et al. 2002) (Khorasani et al. 2008; Wibbenmeyer et al.

2006) and level 3 evidence (Chim et al. 2007; Lari and Alaghehbandan 2000), and supported by Agnihotri et al. (2004), Ozumba and Jiburum (2000) and Singh et al. (2003) at level 4 within Phillips et al.'s (2001) hierarchy of evidence. Current best evidence regarding the likeliest Gram-negative bacteriological profile against which antimicrobial therapy should be targeted not only provides a robust and valid rationale to inform the burns clinician's 'best guess' initial empirical treatment but may also inform Gram-negative BWI treatment in developing countries where over 75% of patients with burn wound infections do not afford the cost of a single wound swab investigation, as illustrated by Komolafe et al. (2003), and Ozumba and Jiburum (2000).

Current best evidence suggests that the incidence of Gram-negative BWI is significantly increased in terror attack victims, with a significantly increased incidence of Acinetobacter BWI. A lower threshold for suspicion and treatment may therefore be feasible. These terror attack victims involved in terrorist attacks may be treated with other 'routine' admissions at civilian institutions which may be subject to clinical performance audit. Therefore, another important implication is that such a patient group could significantly skew the results of such audits regarding infection rates, if they are included without any clarification, when in reality, disparities in their mode of injury; transport and treatment suggest that they may form a separate sub-population in terms of their susceptibility to infection.

Furthermore the standardised incidence rates reported in this study have addressed a gap in the literature, and allowed reflection on the prominent incidence of BWI caused by the Gram-negative BWI profile identified. This contributes to improve awareness of these infections, which are not as publicised as MRSA (BBC 2009) and may also help argue the case for resource-allocation to development of new antimicrobial agents. This is significant considering that out of 506 new FDA-approved pharmaceutical products in the last 10 years; only six were antimicrobials (McConnel 2006; Spellberg et al. 2004).

A significant association between TBSA (Appelgren et al. 2002; Wibbenmeyer et al. 2006), ABSI (Appelgren et al. 2002), increased admission APACHE (II) scores (Wong et al. 2002), LOS (Appelgren et al. 2002; Chim et al. 2007; Mayhall 2003; 2005) , and communal shower therapy (Akin and Ozcan 2003; Church et al. 2006; Mayhall 2003; Simor et al. 2002; Weber and McManus 2004) was underscored by compelling evidence in the literature. Current best evidence also supported TBSA, procedures in communal shower facilities (Simor et al. 2002), and length of stay before isolation, as significant predictive factors for Gram-negative BWI in hospitalised civilian adults. Sufficient evidence therefore supports a grade C recommendation that presence of these factors in a patient's history would be included as part of a risk-assessment process to identify hospitalised civilian adult patients having multiple associations to increased incidence of Gram-negative burn wound infection. Where access to resources that reduce risk of infection is limited, the presence of these associations may provide a robust and valid foundation for resource distribution in cases of limited supply.

Procedures in common shower therapy rooms were identified by Simor et al. (2002) as a significant risk factor for increased incidence of Gram-negative burn wound infection in hospitalised civilian adults. Current best evidence strongly suggest this predictive factor to be associated with the largest magnitude of effect (OR=4.1 at p<0.02). It is recommended that procedures in common shower therapy rooms should be avoided or that disposable sterilised ethylene sheets should be used between patients to prevent contact with fomites as suggested by Akin and Ozcan (2003). Shower therapy superseded immersion hydrotherapy because of the perceived reduction of the risk of infection (rationale, p. 4). Communal shower facilities are still used in mainstream local practice. While a change to individual use facilities is supported by the evidence, this may not always be possible, due to financial constraints such that use of disposable interfaces between patients (such as polythene sheets) is a cheap and practical potential solution supported by current best evidence.

Current best evidence suggests that High TBSA; increased ABSI; Admission APACHE (II) scores; communal shower therapy; LOS should be included as exploratory variables in the investigation of logistic regression model building for predictors of Gram-negative BWI in hospitalised civilian adults. The robustness of the evidence underscoring these factors, the strength of association on univariate and multivariate analysis, and their magnitude of effect form a robust basis for suggesting these factors as exploratory variables for logistical regression model building. Models of predictive variables for Gram-negative BWI in hospitalised civilian adults would constitute powerful tools to identify patients at risk and enable focusing of available resources.

Weber and McManus (2004) Polavarapu's (2008) and Appelgren et al. (2002) observed an increased occurrence of BWI with presence of FTSB, and although Wong et al. (2002) concluded that burn depth was statistically associated to the risk of multiresistant Acinetobacter BWI by univariate analysis their chosen p value (p<0.10) was high increasing risk of type 1 error. Therefore although current best evidence favoured the possibility that burn wound depth may be associated to an increased incidence of Gram-negative BWI in hospitalised civilian adults, further robust evidence may be required to underpin its inclusion in recommendations and this needs to be addressed by future research.

Finally, compelling evidence (Appelgren et al. 2002; Church et al. 2006; Greenhalgh et al. 2007; Wibbenmeyer et al. 2006) suggested the need for standardised, best-evidence criteria for diagnosis of burn wound infection. A critical appraisal analysis and synthesis of the evidence suggests that Greenhalgh et al.'s (2007) criteria constitute current best evidence. These diagnostic definitions are therefore recommended for clinical bedside use and infection surveillance, to reduce over-prescription of antimicrobials and increase concordance between burn surgeons, and burn infection control specialists.

In conclusion, although published studies on Gram-negative BWI are sparse and varied in terms of the quality of the evidence, this study has made it possible to develop graded recommendations for local practice based on a synthesis of the reviewed literature. It has underlined the significance for implementing these recommendations to improve clinical practice in the initial management of Gram negative wound infections. The study has contributed to raising awareness of procedural issues in the initial management of BWI and informing the local setting and colleagues on the aetiology, incidence and specific risk factors for Gram-negative burn wound infection based on current best evidence. The process of evaluating the evidence has highlighted the need for more research focus on BWI and improved methodological rigour.

References

Abbassi, M. et al. 2006. Evaluation of the 10th External Quality Assessment Scheme results in clinical microbiology laboratories in Tehran and districts. *East Mediterr Health J* 12(3-4), pp. 310-315.

Agnihotri, N. et al. 2004. Aerobic bacterial isolates from burn wound infections and their antibiograms--a five-year study. *Burns* 30(3), pp. 241-243.

Akin, S. and Ozcan, M. 2003. Using a plastic sheet to prevent the risk of contamination of the burn wound during the shower. *Burns* 29(3), pp. 280-283.

Albrecht, M. C. et al. 2006. Impact of Acinetobacter infection on the mortality of burn patients. *J Am Coll Surg* 203(4), pp. 546-550.

Altoparlak, U. et al. 2004. The time-related changes of antimicrobial resistance patterns and predominant bacterial profiles of burn wounds and body flora of burned patients. *Burns* 30(7), pp. 660-664.

Ansermino, M. and Hemsley, C. 2004. Intensive care management and control of infection. *BMJ* 329(7459), pp. 220-223.

Appelgren, P. et al. 2002. A prospective study of infections in burn patients. *Burns* 28(1), pp. 39-46.

Armitage, P. et al. 2002. *Statistical Methods in Medical Research.* Massachusetts, US: Blackwell Publishing Co.

Armour, A. D. et al. 2007. The impact of nosocomially-acquired resistant Pseudomonas aeruginosa infection in a burn unit. *J Trauma* 63(1), pp. 164-171.

Babik, J. et al. 2008. Acinetobacter-- serious danger for burn patients. *Acta Chir Plast* 50(1), pp. 27-32.

Baker, R. A. et al. 1996. Degree of burn, location of burn, and length of hospital stay as predictors of psychosocial status and physical functioning. *J Burn Care Rehabil* 17(4), pp. 327-333.

Barret, E. et al. 2005. *Advanced Burns Life Support Provider Manual* Chicago, Illinois, US: American Burns Association.

Barret, J. P. and Herndon, D. N. 2003. Effects of burn wound excision on bacterial colonization and invasion. *Plast Reconstr Surg* 111(2), pp. 744-750; discussion 751-742.

BBC. 2009. MRSA 'not the only threat to NHS' *BBc news* [online], 10 Nov 2009. Available at: <URL: http://news.bbc.co.uk/1/hi/health/8351269.stm> [Accessed: 1 December 2009].

Boucher, H. W. et al. 2009. Bad bugs, no drugs: no ESKAPE! An update from the Infectious Diseases Society of America. *Clin Infect Dis* 48(1), pp. 1-12.

BSAC. 2009. *Burn Wound Infection.* Available at: <URL: http://www.bsac.org.uk/pyxis/Skin%20and%20soft%20tissue%20infections/Burn%20wound %20infection/Burn%20wound%20infection.htm#Aetiology> [Accessed: 31 October 2009].

Calum, H. et al. 2009. Thermal injury induces impaired function in polymorphonuclear neutrophil granulocytes and reduced control of burn wound infection. *Clin Exp Immunol* 156(1), pp. 102-110.

Campbell, M. 2001. *Statistics at Square Two- Understanding Modern Statistical Applciations in Medicine.* First Ed. ed. London: BMJ Publishing Group.

Cardany, C. R. et al. 1985. Influence of hydrotherapy and antiseptic agents on burn wound bacterial contamination. *J Burn Care Rehabil* 6(3), pp. 230-232.

CDC 2001. National Nosocomial Infections Surveillance (NNIS) System Report, Data Summary from January 1992-June 2001, issued August 2001. *Am J Infect Control* 29(6), pp. 404-421.

Ceri, H. et al. 1999. The Calgary Biofilm Device: new technology for rapid determination of antibiotic susceptibilities of bacterial biofilms. *J Clin Microbiol* 37(6), pp. 1771-1776.

Chalise, P. R. et al. 2008. Epidemiological and bacteriological profile of burn patients at Nepal Medical College Teaching Hospital. *Nepal Med Coll J* 10(4), pp. 233-237.

Chim, H. and Song, C. 2007. Aeromonas infection in critically ill burn patients. *Burns* 33(6), pp. 756-759.

Chim, H. et al. 2007. Five-year review of infections in a burn intensive care unit: High incidence of Acinetobacter baumannii in a tropical climate. *Burns* 33(8), pp. 1008-1014.

Church, D. et al. 2006. Burn wound infections. *Clin Microbiol Rev* 19(2), pp. 403-434.

Clark, N. M. et al. 2003. Antimicrobial resistance among gram-positive organisms in the intensive care unit. *Curr Opin Crit Care* 9(5), pp. 403-412.

Crombie, I. 2008. *A Pocket Guide to Critical Appraisal.* Dundee: BMJ Publishing Group.

D'Avignon, L. C. et al. 2008. Prevention and management of infections associated with burns in the combat casualty. *J Trauma* 64(3 Suppl), pp. S277-286.

Dahiya, P. 2009. Burns as a model of SIRS. *Front Biosci* 14, pp. 4962-4967.

Dancey, C. and Reidy, J. 2004. *Statsitics Without Numbers.* 4th Edition ed. Essex: Essex Publishing.

Das, A. and Kim, K. S. 2000. Infections in burn injury. *Pediatr Infect Dis J* 19(8), pp. 737-738.

Dawes, M. et al. 2005. Sicily statement on evidence-based practice. *BMC Med Educ* 5(1), p.

1.

Dougherty, W. and Waxman, K. 1996. The complexities of managing severe burns with associated trauma. *Surg Clin North Am* 76(4), pp. 923-958.

Duncan, R. 2003. The dawning era of polymer therapeutics. *Nat Rev Drug Discov* 2(5), pp. 347-360.

Ebell, M. 1999. Information at the point of care: answering clinical questions. *J Am Board Fam Pract* 12(3), pp. 225-235.

Edwards-Jones, V. and Greenwood, J. E. 2003. What's new in burn microbiology? James Laing Memorial Prize Essay 2000. *Burns* 29(1), pp. 15-24.

Ekrami, A. and Kalantar, E. 2007. Bacterial infections in burn patients at a burn hospital in Iran. *Indian J Med Res* 126(6), pp. 541-544.

Erol, S. et al. 2004. Changes of microbial flora and wound colonization in burned patients. *Burns* 30(4), pp. 357-361.

Estahbanati, H. K. et al. 2002. Frequency of Pseudomonas aeruginosa serotypes in burn wound infections and their resistance to antibiotics. *Burns* 28(4), pp. 340-348.

Evans, D. 2003. Hierarchy of evidence: a framework for ranking evidence evaluating healthcare interventions. *J Clin Nurs* 12(1), pp. 77-84.

Falk, P. S. et al. 2000. Outbreak of vancomycin-resistant enterococci in a burn unit. *Infect Control Hosp Epidemiol* 21(9), pp. 575-582.

Ferreira, A. C. et al. 2004. Emergence of resistance in Pseudomonas aeruginosa and Acinetobacter species after the use of antimicrobials for burned patients. *Infect Control Hosp Epidemiol* 25(10), pp. 868-872.

Flattau, A. et al. 2008. Antibiotic-resistant gram-negative bacteria in deep tissue cultures. *Int Wound J* 5(5), pp. 599-600.

Forbes, B. et al. 1998. *Bailley and Scott's diagnostic microbiology*. St. Louis: Mosby, p. .

Gales, A. C. et al. 2001. Emerging importance of multidrug-resistant Acinetobacter species and Stenotrophomonas maltophilia as pathogens in seriously ill patients: geographic patterns, epidemiological features, and trends in the SENTRY Antimicrobial Surveillance Program (1997-1999). *Clin Infect Dis* 32 Suppl 2, pp. S104-113.

Gallagher, J. 2009. *USA data on Burn Wound Infection in Hospitalised Civilian Adults-Personal Correspondence.* to: Azzopardi, E. Received November 2009.

Garner, J. S. et al. 1988. CDC definitions for nosocomial infections, 1988. *Am J Infect Control* 16(3), pp. 128-140.

Geyik, M. F. et al. 2003. Epidemiology of burn unit infections in children. *Am J Infect*

Control 31(6), pp. 342-346.

Gomez, R. et al. 2009. Causes of mortality by autopsy findings of combat casualties and civilian patients admitted to a burn unit. *J Am Coll Surg* 208(3), pp. 348-354.

Gray, M. and Meakins, J. L. 2006. Evidence-based surgical practice and patient-centered care: inevitable. *Surg Clin North Am* 86(1), pp. 217-220.

Greenhalgh, D. G. et al. 2007. American Burn Association consensus conference to define sepsis and infection in burns. *J Burn Care Res* 28(6), pp. 776-790.

Greenhalgh, T. 2001. *How to Read a Paper- the Basics of Evidence Based Medicine*. Third Edition ed. London: BMJ Publishing Group.

Greenwood, D. et al. 2002. *Medical Microbiology*. 16th Ed. ed. Nottingham: Churchill Livingstone.

Guggenheim, M. et al. 2009. Changes in bacterial isolates from burn wounds and their antibiograms: A 20-year study (1986-2005). *Burns* (of Publication: June 2009), pp. 35(34)(pp 553-560), 2009.

Harrison-Balestra, C. et al. 2003. A wound-isolated Pseudomonas aeruginosa grows a biofilm in vitro within 10 hours and is visualized by light microscopy. *Dermatol Surg* 29(6), pp. 631-635.

Herndon, D. N. 1996. *Total Burn Care*. 3rd Edition ed. Philadelphia, USA: Elsevier.

Herndon, D. N. 2009. *Data regarding Aetiology, Incidence and Risk Factors for Hospital Acquired Burn Wound Infection in Adult Civilian Patients (Personal Communication)*. to: Azzopardi, E. Received 31 October 2009.

Herruzo, R. et al. 2004. Two consecutive outbreaks of Acinetobacter baumanii 1-a in a burn Intensive Care Unit for adults. *Burns* (of Publication: Aug 2004), pp. 30(35)(pp 419-423), 2004.

Hodle, A. E. et al. 2006. Infection control practices in U.S. burn units. *J Burn Care Res* 27(2), pp. 142-151.

Horan, T. C. et al. 2008. CDC/NHSN surveillance definition of health care-associated infection and criteria for specific types of infections in the acute care setting. *Am J Infect Control* 36(5), pp. 309-332.

Huang, K. L. et al. 2008. Systemic inflammation caused by white smoke inhalation in a combat exercise. *Chest* 133(3), pp. 722-728.

Huang, X. et al. 2006. Evaluation of PICO as a knowledge representation for clinical questions. *AMIA Annu Symp Proc*, pp. 359-363.

Ipaktchi, K. et al. 2006. Attenuating burn wound inflammatory signaling reduces systemic inflammation and acute lung injury. *J Immunol* 177(11), pp. 8065-8071.

Jadad, A. 1998. *Randomised Controlled Trials*. London: BMJ Publishing.

Japoni, A. et al. 2009. Pseudomonas aeruginosa: Burn infection, treatment and antibacterial resistance. *Iranian Red Crescent Medical Journal* (of Publication: 2009), pp. 11(13)(pp 244-253), 2009.

Jewell, N. 2004. *Statistics for Epidemiology*. US: Chapman Hall/CRC.

Kaushik, R. et al. 2001. Bacteriology of burn wounds--the first three years in a new burn unit at the Medical College Chandigarh. *Burns* 27(6), pp. 595-597.

Kauvar, D. S. et al. 2006. Comparison of combat and non-combat burns from ongoing U.S. military operations. *J Surg Res* 132(2), pp. 195-200.

Khorasani, G. et al. 2008. Profile of microorganisms and antimicrobial resistance at a tertiary care referral burn centre in Iran: emergence of Citrobacter freundii as a common microorganism. *Burns* 34(7), pp. 947-952.

Komolafe, O. O. et al. 2003. Bacteriology of burns at the Queen Elizabeth Central Hospital, Blantyre, Malawi. *Burns* 29(3), pp. 235-238.

Lari, A. R. and Alaghehbandan, R. 2000. Nosocomial infections in an Iranian burn care center. *Burns* 26(8), pp. 737-740.

Maragakis, L. L. and Perl, T. M. 2008. Acinetobacter baumannii: epidemiology, antimicrobial resistance, and treatment options. *Clin Infect Dis* 46(8), pp. 1254-1263.

Mason, A. D., Jr. et al. 1986. Association of burn mortality and bacteremia. A 25-year review. *Arch Surg* 121(9), pp. 1027-1031.

Mayer, D. 2004. *Essential Evidence Based Medicine*. 1 ed. Cambridge: Cambridge University Press.

Mayhall, C. G. 2003. The epidemiology of burn wound infections: then and now. *Clin Infect Dis* 37(4), pp. 543-550.

McConnel, J. 2006. The future should not look like the past. *Lancet Infect Dis* 6(5), p. 253.

McDonald, L. C. et al. 1999. Seasonal variation of Acinetobacter infections: 1987-1996. Nosocomial Infections Surveillance System. *Clin Infect Dis* 29(5), pp. 1133-1137.

McMillian, J. and Schumacher, S. 1997. *Research in education: A conceptual introduction* NV, USA: Addison Weseley.

Meyer, D. 2004. *Essential Evidence Based Medicine*. 1 ed. Cambridge: Cambridge University Press.

Miranda, B. H. et al. 2008. Two stage study of wound microorganisms affecting burns and plastic surgery inpatients. *J Burn Care Res* 29(6), pp. 927-932.

Moissenet, D. et al. 2000. Nosocomial Infections in Pediatric Patients with Burns Results of a Prospective Study Over One Year. In: *Intersci Conf Antimicrob Agents Chemother*. Paris. p. 414.

Mshana, S. E. et al. 2009. Prevalence of multiresistant gram-negative organisms in a tertiary hospital in Mwanza, Tanzania. *BMC Res Notes* 2, p. 49.

Nasser, S. et al. 2003. Colonization of burn wounds in Ain Shams University Burn Unit. *Burns* (of Publication: May 2003), pp. 29(23)(pp 229-233), 2003.

Nelson, R. 2003. Antibiotic development pipeline runs dry. New drugs to fight resistant organisms are not being developed, experts say. *Lancet* 362(9397), pp. 1726-1727.

Newman, M. and Roberts, T. 2002. *Critical Appraisal: Is the quality of the study good enough for you to use the findings? In Craig JV, Smyth RL. (Eds). The Evidence Based Practice Manual for Nurses*. Edinburgh: Churchill Livingstone.

NLM. 2009. *MeSH Browser (2010 MeSH)*. [Internet Website]. Available at: <URL: [Accessed: 27 September 2009].

Oncul, O. et al. 2002. The evaluation of nosocomial infection during 1-year-period in the burn unit of a training hospital in Istanbul, Turkey. *Burns* 28(8), pp. 738-744.

Ozkurt, Z. et al. 2005. The risk factors for acquisition of imipenem-resistant Pseudomonas aeruginosa in the burn unit. *Burns* 31(7), pp. 870-873.

Ozumba, U. C. and Jiburum, B. C. 2000. Bacteriology of burn wounds in Enugu, Nigeria. *Burns* 26(2), pp. 178-180.

Peck, M. D. et al. 1998. Surveillance of burn wound infections: a proposal for definitions. *J Burn Care Rehabil* 19(5), pp. 386-389.

Perencevich, E. N. et al. 2008. Summer Peaks in the Incidences of Gram-Negative Bacterial Infection Among Hospitalized Patients. *Infect Control Hosp Epidemiol* 29(12), pp. 1124-1131.

Phillips, P. et al. 2001. *Oxford Centre for Evidence-based Medicine - Levels of Evidence (March 2009)*. [Internet Web page]. University of Oxford. Available at: <URL: [Accessed: 1st September 2009].

Polavarapu, N. et al. 2008. Microbiology of burn wound infections. *J Craniofac Surg* 19(4), pp. 899-902.

Polit, D. et al. 2006. *Nursing Research: Methods Appraisal and Utilization*. 5th Edition ed. Philadelphia: Lipincott Williams & Wilkins.

Public Health Resource Unit, E. 2006. *Critical Appraisal Skills Program (CASP) making sense of evidence, 10 questions to help you make sense of qualitative research*. Oxford Univsristy. Available at: <URL: [Accessed: 1st September 2009].

Ram, S. et al. 2000. Prevalence of multidrug resistant organisms in an intensive care burn unit. *Indian J Med Res* 111, pp. 118-120.

Rees, C. 2004. *An introduction to research for midwives*. Cardiff: Elsevier Health

Rees, C. and Taylor, A. 2001. Module 1 Research.*MSc Advanced Surgical Practice Modules*. Cardiff: p. 33.

Richardson, W. S. et al. 1995. The well-built clinical question: a key to evidence-based decisions. *ACP J Club* 123(3), pp. A12-13.

Rodgers, G. L. et al. 2000. Predictors of infectious complications after burn injuries in children. *Pediatr Infect Dis J* 19(10), pp. 990-995.

Sackett, D. L. and Rosenberg, W. M. 1995. The need for evidence-based medicine. *J R Soc Med* 88(11), pp. 620-624.

Sackett, D. L. et al. 1996. Evidence based medicine: what it is and what it isn't. *BMJ* 312(7023), pp. 71-72.

Santucci, S. G. et al. 2003. Infections in a burn intensive care unit: Experience of seven years. *Journal of Hospital Infection* (of Publication: Jan 2003), pp. 53(51)(pp 56-13), 2003.

Sheridan, R. L. et al. 1993. Flavobacterial sepsis in massively burned pediatric patients. *Clinical Infectious Diseases* (of Publication: 1993), pp. 17(12)(pp 185-187), 1993.

Silla, R. C. et al. 2006. Infection in acute burn wounds following the Bali bombings: a comparative prospective audit. *Burns* 32(2), pp. 139-144.

Simor, A. E. et al. 2002. An outbreak due to multiresistant Acinetobacter baumannii in a burn unit: risk factors for acquisition and management. *Infect Control Hosp Epidemiol* 23(5), pp. 261-267.

Singh, N. P. et al. 2003. Changing trends in bacteriology of burns in the burns unit, Delhi, India. *Burns* 29(2), pp. 129-132.

Sokal, R. and Rohlf, F. 1981. *Biometry: The Principles and Practice of Statistics in Biological Research*. Oxford: Oxford University Press.

Song, W. et al. 2001. Microbiologic aspects of predominant bacteria isolated from the burn patients in Korea. *Burns* 27(2), pp. 136-139.

Spellberg, B. et al. 2004. Trends in Antimicrobial Drug Development: Implications for the Future. *Antimicrobial Research & Development* 38(1), pp. 1279-1285.

Strauss, S. et al. 2005. Evidence Based Medicine 3rd Edition.

Swinscow, T. and Campbell, M. 2002. *Statistics at Square One*. 10th Edition ed. London: BMJ Publishing Group.

Tredget, E. E. et al. 2004. Pseudomonas infections in the thermally injured patient. *Burns* 30(1), pp. 3-26.

Uppal, S. K. et al. 2007. Comparative evaluation of surface swab and quantitative full thickness wound biopsy culture in burn patients. *Burns* 33(4), pp. 460-463.

Weber, J. and McManus, A. 2004. Infection control in burn patients. *Burns* 30(8), pp. A16-24.

Wente, M. N. et al. 2003. Perspectives of evidence-based surgery. *Dig Surg* 20(4), pp. 263-269.

Wibbenmeyer, L. et al. 2006. Prospective analysis of nosocomial infection rates, antibiotic use, and patterns of resistance in a burn population. *J Burn Care Res* 27(2), pp. 152-160.

Wong, T. H. et al. 2002. Multi-resistant Acinetobacter baumannii on a burns unit--clinical risk factors and prognosis. *Burns* 28(4), pp. 349-357.

Yildirim, S. et al. 2005. Bacteriological profile and antibiotic resistance: Comparison of findings in a burn intensive care unit, other intensive care units, and the hospital services unit of a single center. *Journal of Burn Care and Rehabilitation* (of Publication: Nov 2005), pp. 26(26)(pp 488-492), 2005.

Yousefi-Mashouf, R. and Hashemi, S. H. 2006. The epidemiology of burn wound infections in patients hospitalized in burn center of Hamedan, Western Iran. *Journal of Medical Sciences* (of Publication: May 2006), pp. 6(3)(pp 426-431), 2006.

Appendix

Appendix 1: Excluded Studies

	Excluded Studies	
	Study	Reason
1	Das &Kim (2000)	Paediatric population; does not inform the aims
2	Santucci et al. (2003)	Paediatric population; does not inform the aims
3	Geyik et al. (2003)	Paediatric population; does not inform the aims
4	Rodgers et al. (2000)	Paediatric population; does not inform the aims
5	Ferreira et al. (2004)	Paediatric population; does not inform the aims
6	Song et al. (2001)	Paediatric population; does not inform the aims
7	Ekrami & Kalantar (2007)	Study included data from BWI and other sources of infection such that the results could not inform the terms of reference
8	Falk et al. (2000)	The study population was due to diarrhoea in a burn unit not BWI. Therefore the results could not inform the aim
9	Albrecht et al. (2006)	The paper was used to inform the critical appraisal, but its aims did not inform the terms of reference as it only sought to determine the risk of mortality of Acinetobacter infection
10	Japoni et al. (2009)	Not relevant to the terms of reference
11	Nasser et al. (2003)	The authors investigate colonisation not BWI
12	Yildrim et al (2005)	Includes paediatric and neonatal individuals in the sample
13	(2004)	Sample population is not exclusively limited to adults and the results for adults cannot be separately interpreted.
14	Guggenheim e al. (2009)	The study centres purely on colonisation not infection hence does not inform the terms of reference
15	Yousefi-Mashouf & Hashemi (2006)	Data includes children as the commonest age group.
16	Estahbanati et al. (2002)	Study sample does not specifically address an adult population
17	Chalise et al. (2008)	Study includes children and adults, aetiology or incidences nor risk factors are described despite title
18	Miranda et al. (2008)	Study included military subjects
19	Falk et al. (2000)	Study does not differentiate between infection and colonisation or contamination
20	Erol et al. (2004)	Study specifically addressed colonisation
21	Herruzo et al. (2004)	Study addressed prevalence rather than incidence rates and hence could not inform the study

Appendix 2:
Rees' (1997) Framework for Critical Appraisal of Quantitative Research

Focus: In broad terms what is the theme of the article? What are the key words you would file this under? Are the key words in the title a clue to the focus? How important s this focus for clinical practice?
Background: What argument or evidence does the researcher provide that suggests his topic is worth exploring? Is there a critical review of previous research on the subject? Are local problems or changes that justify the study presented? Is there a trigger that answers the question: Why did they do it?
Terms of Reference: Does the researcher state the terms of reference? In the case of clinical research there may be only a statement of hypothesis that the researcher wished to test. Is it possible to identify dependent and independent variables? Remember level one questions will not have both neither will a correlation study. Are there concepts and operational definitions?
Study design: What is the broad research approach? Is it experimental is it descriptive? Is it action research or audit? Is it quantitative or qualitative? Is the study design appropriate to the terms of reference / hypothesis / research question?
Data collection methods: What tool of data collection has been used? Has a single method been used or triangulation? Has the author addressed issues of reliability and validity? Has a pilot study been conducted? Have strengths and limitations been recognised by the author?
Ethical considerations: Were the issues of informed consent and confidentiality addressed? Was any harm or discomfort to individuals balanced against benefits? Did a local ethics committee consider the study?
Sample: Who or what made up the sample? Were there clear inclusion and exclusion criteria? What method of sampling was used? Are those in the sample typical and representative or are there any obvious elements of bias? On how many sample units are the results based?
Data presentation: In what from are the results presented? Does the author explain and comment on these? Has the author used correlation to establish whether certain variables are associated with each other? Have tests of significance been used to establish to what extent any differences between groups and variables are could have happened by chance? Can sense be made of the way the results have been presented or could the author have provided more explanation
Main findings: What are the most important results that relate to the term of reference /hypothesis/ research question?
Conclusions and recommendations: What is the answer to the terms of reference /research question? If relevant was the hypothesis accepted or rejected? Are the conclusions made based on and supported by the results? What recommendations are made for practice? Are these relevant feasible or specific?
Readability: How easy is it to read? Is it written in a clear interesting style of a heavy style? Does it assume a great deal of technical knowledge about the subject or research procedures?
Practical Implications: How could the results be related to practice? Who might find it relevant and in what way? What questions does it pose for practice and further study?

Source: Framework for Critiquing Quantitative Research (after Rees C, 1997), Cited in Rees C, Taylor A, (2007) Module 1A –Research, Cardiff University October 2007 (Page 35 Table 5A)

Appendix 3:
Framework for critical appraisal of qualitative research Public Health Research Unit (2006)

---

1. Was there a clear statement of the aims of the research? Consider:
– what the goal of the research was - why it is important – its relevance

2. Is a qualitative methodology appropriate? Consider:

– if the research seeks to interpret or illuminate the actions and/or subjective experiences of research participants

---

Detailed questions

Appropriate research design

3. Was the research design appropriate to address the aims of the research? Consider:
   – if the researcher has justified the research design (e.g. have they discussed how they   decided which methods to use?)

Sampling

4. Was the recruitment strategy appropriate to the aims of the research? Consider:
   – if the researcher has explained how the participants were selected
   – if they explained why the participants they selected were the most appropriate to provide access to the type of knowledge sought by the study
   – if there are any discussions around recruitment (e.g. why some people chose not to take part)

Data collection

5. Were the data collected in a way that addressed the research issue? Consider:
   – if the setting for data collection was justified

   – if it is clear how data were collected (e.g. focus group, semi-structured interview etc)
   – if the researcher has justified the methods chosen
   – if the researcher has made the methods explicit (e.g. for interview method, is there an indication
   of how interviews were conducted, did they use a topic guide?)
   – if methods were modified during the study. If so, has the researcher explained how and why?
   – if the form of data is clear (e.g. tape recordings, video material, notes etc)
   – if the researcher has discussed saturation of   data

Reflexivity (research partnership relations/recognition of researcher bias)

6. Has the relationship between researcher and participants been adequately considered?
   Consider whether it is clear:

– if the researcher critically examined their own role, potential bias and influence during: formulation of research questions and data collection, including sample recruitment   and choice of location
– how the researcher responded to events during the study and whether they considered the implications of any changes in the research design

---

Appendix 3- Continued
Framework for critical appraisal of qualitative research Public Health Research Unit (2006)

Ethical Issues

7. Have ethical issues been taken into consideration? Consider:

– if there are sufficient details of how the research was explained to participants for the reader to assess whether ethical standards were maintained if the researcher has discussed issues raised by the study (e. g. issues around informed consent or confidentiality or how they have handled the effects of the study on the participants during and after the study)
- if approval has been sought from the ethics committee

Data Analysis

8. Was the data analysis sufficiently rigorous? *Consider:*

– *if there is an in-depth description of the analysis   process*
– *if thematic analysis is used. If so, is it clear how the categories/themes were derived from the data?*
– *whether the researcher explains how the data presented were selected from the original*
  sample to demonstrate the analysis process

– *if sufficient data are presented to support the findings*
– *to what extent contradictory data are taken into account*
– *whether the researcher critically examined their own role, potential bias and influence during*
  analysis and selection of data for presentation

Findings

9. Is there a clear statement of findings? *Consider:*

– *if the findings are explicit*

– *if there is adequate discussion of the evidence both for and against the researcher's arguments*
– *if the researcher has discussed the credibility of their findings (e.g. triangulation, respondent*
  Validation, more than one analyst.)

– *if the findings are discussed in relation to the original research questions*

Value of the research

10. How valuable is the research? *Consider:*

– *If the researcher discusses the contribution the study makes to existing knowledge or understanding (e.g. do they consider the findings in relation to current practice or policy, or relevant research-based literature?)*
– *if they identify new areas where research is necessary*
– *if the researchers have discussed whether or how the findings can be transferred to other populations or*
    considered other ways the research may be used

Source: Public Health Research Unit (2006) Critical Appraisal Skills Programme
(CASP): making sense of the evidence

Appendix 4:
Framework for critical appraisal of narrative reviews. (McMillian and Schumacher 1997)

A narrative literature review is judged by three criteria: its selection of the sources, its criticism of the literature; and its summary and overall interpretation of the literature on the problem. Below are questions that aid a reader in determining the quality of the literature review.

Selection of the Literature

1. Is the purpose of the review (preliminary or exhaustive) indicated?

2. Are the parameters of the review reasonable?
a. Why were certain bodies of literature included in the search and others excluded from it?
b. Which years were included in the search?

3. Is the primary literature emphasised in the review and secondary literature, if cited, used selectively?

4. Are recent developments in the problem emphasised in the review?

5. Is the literature selected relevant to the problem?

6. Are complete bibliographic data provided for each reference?

Criticism of the Literature

1. Is the review organised by topics or ideas, not by author?

2. Is the review organised logically?

3. Are major studies or theories discussed in detail and minor studies with similar limitations or results discussed as a group?

4. Is there adequate criticism of the design and methodology of important studies so that the reader can draw his or her own conclusions?

5. Are studies compared and contrasted and conflicting or inconclusive results noted?

6. Is the relevance of each reference to the problem explicit?

Summary & Interpretation

1. Does the summary provide an overall interpretation and understanding of our knowledge of the problem?

2. Do the implications provide theoretical or empirical justification for the specific research questions or hypotheses to follow?

3. Do the methodological implications provide a rationale for the design to follow?

Source: McMillian, J. and Schumacher, S. (1997). *Research in education: A conceptual introduction* (4th edition), pp. 152-153-308. NY: HarpersCollins College Publishers.

Appendix 5:
Hierarchy of Evidence Levels and Grades of Recommendations (Phillips et al. 2001)

Level	Therapy /Prevention, Aetiology/Harm	Prognosis	Diagnosis	Differential diagnosis/symptom prevalence study	Economic and decision analyses
1a	SR (with homogeneity*) of RCTs	SR (with homogeneity*) of inception cohort studies; CDR† validated in different populations	SR (with homogeneity*) of Level 1 diagnostic studies; CDR† with 1b studies	SR (with homogeneity*) of prospective cohort studies	SR (with homogeneity*) of Level 1 economic studies
1b	Individual RCT (with narrow Confidence Interval‡)	Individual inception cohort study with > 80% follow-up; CDR† validated in a single population	Validating** cohort study with good††† reference standards; or CDR† tested within one clinical centre	Prospective cohort study with good follow-up****	Analysis based on clinically sensible costs or alternatives; systematic review(s) of the evidence; and including multi-way sensitivity analyses
1c	All or none§	All or none case-series	Absolute SpPins and SnNouts††	All or none case-series	Absolute better-value or worse-value analyses ††††
2a	SR (with homogeneity*) of cohort studies	SR (with homogeneity*) of either retrospective cohort studies or untreated control groups in RCTs	SR (with homogeneity*) of Level >2 diagnostic studies	SR (with homogeneity*) of 2b and better studies	SR (with homogeneity*) of Level >2 economic studies
2b	Individual cohort study (including low quality RCT; e.g., <80% follow-up)	Retrospective cohort study or follow-up of untreated control patients in an RCT; Derivation of CDR† or validated on split-sample§§§ only	Exploratory** cohort study with good††† reference standards; CDR† after derivation, or validated only on split-sample§§§ or databases	Retrospective cohort study, or poor follow-up	Analysis based on clinically sensible costs or alternatives; limited review(s) of the evidence, or single studies; and including multi-way sensitivity analyses
2c	"Outcomes" Research; Ecological studies	"Outcomes" Research		Ecological studies	Audit or outcomes research
3a	SR (with homogeneity*) of case-control studies		SR (with homogeneity*) of 3b and better studies	SR (with homogeneity*) of 3b and better studies	SR (with homogeneity*) of 3b and better studies
3b	Individual Case-Control Study		Non-consecutive study; or without consistently applied reference standards	Non-consecutive cohort study, or very limited population	Analysis based on limited alternatives or costs, poor quality estimates of data, but including sensitivity analyses incorporating clinically sensible variations.

4	Case-series (and poor quality cohort and case-control studies§§)	Case-series (and poor quality prognostic cohort studies***)	Case-control study, poor or non-independent reference standard	Case-series or superseded reference standards	Analysis with no sensitivity analysis
5	Expert opinion without explicit critical appraisal, or based on physiology, bench research or "first principles"				

Notes Users can add a minus-sign "-" to denote the level of that fails to provide a conclusive answer because: **EITHER** a single result with a wide Confidence Interval **OR** a Systematic Review with troublesome heterogeneity. Such evidence is inconclusive, and therefore can only generate Grade D recommendations.

*	By homogeneity we mean a systematic review that is free of worrisome variations (heterogeneity) in the directions and degrees of results between individual studies. Not all systematic reviews with statistically significant heterogeneity need be worrisome, and not all worrisome heterogeneity need be statistically significant. As noted above, studies displaying worrisome heterogeneity should be tagged with a "-" at the end of their designated level.
†	Clinical Decision Rule. (These are algorithms or scoring systems that lead to a prognostic estimation or a diagnostic category.)
‡	See note above for advice on how to understand, rate and use trials or other studies with wide confidence intervals.
§	Met when all patients died before the Rx became available, but some now survive on it; or when some patients died before the Rx became available, but none now die on it.
§§	By poor quality cohort study we mean one that failed to clearly define comparison groups and/or failed to measure exposures and outcomes in the same (preferably blinded), objective way in both exposed and non-exposed individuals and/or failed to identify or appropriately control known confounders and/or failed to carry out a sufficiently long and complete follow-up of patients. By poor quality case-control study we mean one that failed to clearly define comparison groups and/or failed to measure exposures and outcomes in the same (preferably blinded), objective way in both cases and controls and/or failed to identify or appropriately control known confounders.
§§§	Split-sample validation is achieved by collecting all the information in a single tranche, then artificially dividing this into "derivation" and "validation" samples.
††	An "Absolute SpPin" is a diagnostic finding whose Specificity is so high that a Positive result rules-in the diagnosis. An "Absolute SnNout" is a diagnostic finding whose Sensitivity is so high that a Negative result rules-out the diagnosis.
‡‡	Good, better, bad and worse refer to the comparisons between treatments in terms of their clinical risks and benefits.
†††	Good reference standards are independent of the test, and applied blindly or objectively to applied to all patients. Poor reference standards are haphazardly applied, but still independent of the test. Use of a non-independent reference standard (where the 'test' is included in the 'reference', or where the 'testing' affects the 'reference') implies a level 4 study.
††† †	Better-value treatments are clearly as good but cheaper, or better at the same or reduced cost. Worse-value treatments are as good and more expensive, or worse and the equally or more expensive.
**	Validating studies test the quality of a specific diagnostic test, based on prior evidence. An exploratory study collects information and trawls the data (e.g. using a regression analysis) to find which factors are 'significant'.
***	By poor quality prognostic cohort study we mean one in which sampling was biased in favour of patients who already had the target outcome, or the measurement of outcomes was accomplished in <80% of study patients, or outcomes were determined in an unblinded, non-objective way, or there was no correction for confounding factors.
*** *	Good follow-up in a differential diagnosis study is >80%, with adequate time for alternative diagnoses to emerge (for example 1-6 months acute, 1 - 5 years chronic)

Grades of Recommendation

A	consistent level 1 studies
B	consistent level 2 or 3 studies *or* extrapolations from level 1 studies
C	level 4 studies *or* extrapolations from level 2 or 3 studies
D	level 5 evidence *or* troublingly inconsistent or inconclusive studies of any level

"Extrapolations" are where data is used in a situation that has potentially clinically important differences than the original study situation.

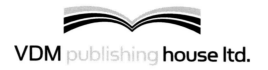
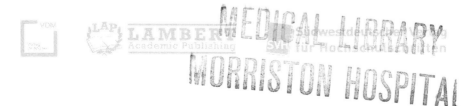